The spiritual journey of a Jewish Christian
The struggle with a crippling disease
A life changing bonding with gulag survivors
                    in post-Soviet Russia

GOD CALLS ME MIRIAM

by
Miriam Elizabeth Stulberg

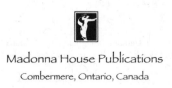
Madonna House Publications
Combermere, Ontario, Canada

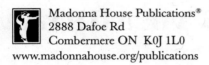

Madonna House Publications®
2888 Dafoe Rd
Combermere ON K0J 1L0
www.madonnahouse.org/publications

God Calls Me Miriam
by Miriam Elizabeth Stulberg

First Edition
First printing, March 25, 2009—Feast of the Annunciation of the Lord

Printed in Canada

Design and layout by Rob Huston

This book is set in Baskerville, created in 1752 by John Baskerville, an English typefounder and printer. Headings are set in Catull, designed by Gustav Jaeger in 1982.

Library and Archives Canada Cataloguing in Publication

Stulberg, Miriam, 1947–

   God calls me Miriam : the spiritual journey of a Jewish Christian : the struggle with a crippling disease : a life changing bonding with Gulag survivors in post-Soviet Russia / Miriam (Mary Beth) Stulberg.

   ISBN 978-1-897145-07-4

   1. Stulberg, Miriam, 1947–. 2. Catholics–Biography. 3. Madonna House (Magadan, Russia)–Biography. 4. Multiple sclerosis–Patients–Biography. 5. Magadan (Russia)–Biography. I. Title.

BX4705.S88A3 2009   282.092   C2009-900419-4

Contents

Preface

Born into an American, liberally-Jewish family, I was baptized as an adult at Madonna House, a Catholic community of laymen, laywomen, and priests, with its centre in Combermere, Ontario, Canada.

I thought the great adventure of my life was over, but I couldn't have been more mistaken. For almost forty years this adventure, this quest for "life in abundance" promised by Christ, has continued unabated, with unforeseen twists and turns and ever-increasing depth and richness. My vocation to Madonna House has been the context for this journey. Its framework has been the spiritual heritage of Catherine de Hueck Doherty, synthesized in what we call the "Little Mandate," and my travelling companions—my brothers and sisters in Madonna House.

In 1992 God brought me to Russia, a land whose history has been forged in the cross and resurrection of Jesus Christ. The following year we opened a house in Magadan, the Russian city most closely associated with Stalin's slave labour camps, and for the next twelve years, my mentors were men and women whose souls had been purified in the crucible of suffering. They gave me a new frame of reference and changed forever the terms in which I understood reality. Because of them, when I was diagnosed with multiple sclerosis in 1998, what might have been an overwhelming blow became instead a new and deeper phase of my spiritual journey.

This book is an attempt to share what the Russian people, and especially the camp survivors, have taught me. I offer these pages in gratitude for the immense privilege of friendship, trust, and love of which I and other members of Madonna House have been the recipients.

While all those mentioned in this book are real people, I have changed many of the names—not only out of sensitivity to the individuals themselves, but also to spare the reader the difficulty of keeping track of five women named Lyuda and a whole bevy of Olgas. In Russian, the use of the patronymic helps to narrow the field, but since most Westerners are unfamiliar with this system, it was simpler to vary the names.

My deep thanks to: Linda Lambeth, director of Madonna House Publications, for her unflagging encouragement and support from the conception of this project to its completion; Réjeanne George, who read each chapter as it was written; Karen Stahl, whose invaluable comments and suggestions guided my revisions; Sylvia Siffary for her constructive criticism, Tom Kluger for his help, and Doreen Chapman, who generously agreed to proofread this manuscript.

Finally, my love and gratitude to Raia Gershzon, her husband Volodya Erokhin, and my goddaughter Masha, with whom we are no longer Russian or American, but simply *rodnyie*–a wonderful Russian word that denotes "family," "one's own."

Miriam Stulberg
Marian Centre
Edmonton, Alberta
March 2009

The Little Mandate[*]

Arise—go! Sell all you possess. Give it directly,
    personally to the poor. Take up my cross (their
    cross) and follow me, going to the poor, being poor,
    being one with them, one with me.

Little—be always little! Be simple, poor, childlike.

Preach the Gospel with your life—without compromise!
    Listen to the Spirit. He will lead you.

Do little things exceedingly well for love of me.

Love...love...love, never counting the cost.

Go into the marketplace and stay with me. Pray, fast.
    Pray always, fast.

Be hidden. Be a light to your neighbour's feet.
    Go without fear into the depths of men's hearts.
    I shall be with you.

Pray always. I will be your rest.

---

[*] Words that Catherine Doherty believed she received from Christ and which express the spirit of the Madonna House Apostolate.

God Calls Me Miriam

One evening in the early 1990s, while I was assigned to Madonna House in Paris, an elderly Frenchwoman invited our staff to dinner. When we had finished dessert, she suggested we browse through her library while she brewed coffee in the kitchen. I was an inveterate book-lover, and nothing could have pleased me more. Scanning the titles on the bookshelves, I came across an old atlas that, upon examination, turned out to have been published at the turn of the century. My heart pounding, I flipped through the pages until I found:

> **Radzivilov:** *A town in European Russia (Volyniya), 37 km west-northwest of Kremenetz on the Slovnia river, near the Austrian border across from Brody in Galicia; 7,350 inhabitants, almost all Jewish. A major customs post.*

It was the first time I'd ever seen a written reference to the place of my family's origin. With his father and older brother, my paternal grandfather, Zalman Stulberg, had left Radzivilov for America in 1908 to escape the anti-Semitic pogroms. They later brought over the rest of the family.

I always regretted not having asked my grandfather about his early life while his memory was still intact. The only discussion I remember occurred when I was sixteen, and he and my grandmother had come to Detroit from their home in Minnesota on their annual visit to our family. I had been playing a record by a Russian-Jewish folk singer and discovered that my grandfather understood some of the Ukrainian lyrics. That's when he told me about Radzivilov.

I couldn't find it on a map. I couldn't even figure out what country it belonged to. My confusion was well justified, for the region of Galicia, where Radzivilov was located, had for centuries been tossed like a football from one nation or empire to another. In my grandfather's time, it had belonged to Austria-Hungary. After World War I it was given to Poland, occupied by the Germans during World War II, liberated by the Soviets, and promptly incorporated into the USSR. Today it is part of an independent Ukraine.

I came across Radzivilov a second time in a short story by Isaac Babel, "The Death of Dolgushov," in his collection *Red Calvary*. Halfway down the first page was the announcement, "Radzivilov is burning!"

Had it been destroyed? Was that why I couldn't find it on a map? No, it still existed, said the Ukrainian bishop I met in Siberia some years later. I told him that my grandfather had been born in what was now his diocese and that I had located the neighbouring town of Brody on a modern map, but not Radzivilov. The bishop thought the town might have been renamed.

All four of my grandparents had immigrated to the United States from Eastern Europe at the beginning of the twentieth century. Zalman's wife, my grandma Mary (anglicized from Miriam), was brought over as a baby from Lithuania. My maternal grandmother, Mary Elizabeth, had been born in Rumania, and she too had originally been called Miriam. She died before I was born, and I was named Mary Beth in her memory.

Karl Danzig, my mother's father, was also a Lithuanian Jew. As a boy of thirteen, he had been forced to leave home to avoid being taken into the Russian army. Conscription at that time meant twenty years of forced service, and most of those unlucky enough to be drafted never returned. An older brother, whom Karl adored, had disappeared some time earlier to escape induction. No one knew where he was, and since it was too risky for Karl to wait, he made his way to Hamburg and boarded a ship to New York, where an uncle was already living. One day on board the ship someone pointed out to the lonely boy another passenger who spoke his language. Approaching him, my grandfather discovered—his missing brother!

Once settled in America, both sets of grandparents, like many other first generation immigrants of that era, shut a psychological door on the Old Country and applied themselves to acquiring a new way of life. My grandfathers joined Conservative synagogues, in which both English and Hebrew were used for prayer and the ritual requirements were adapted to the demands of life in a pluralistic society.* At the age of thirteen, my father and his younger brother each received *bar mitzvah*, the ceremony that marks a Jewish boy's passage into adulthood and allows him to participate fully in the rituals of the synagogue. On reaching chronological adulthood, however, both of them abandoned religious practice.

At home my grandparents stopped speaking Yiddish, except when they didn't want to be understood, and they didn't seem to notice the children's embarrassment at their heavily-accented English. As in most Jewish families, education was a priority. Both my parents were university graduates, and my father and uncle each earned a Ph.D.

When I was two-and-a-half, and my sister Peggy just a baby, my father accepted a position as a microbiologist at the Child Research Center of Michigan, and we moved to Detroit. For the first five years we lived in rented homes in various parts of the city, but shortly after the birth of my brother in 1954, my parents bought a three-bedroom house in the suburb of Oak Park. One factor in their choice was Oak Park's large Jewish population, as they did not want us children to experience the anti-Semitism they had known.

My sister Peggy and I received little formal religious education. For a few months we attended Sunday school at a Conservative synagogue, but our parents pulled us out when we began asking why our family didn't observe the Sabbath and why we ate pork chops at home! When we were very young, my parents would buy a Christmas tree and have us hang up our stockings so that we wouldn't feel different from our Christian friends and neighbours. Later we celebrated both Christmas and Hanukkah (the Jewish Feast of Lights, which also falls in December) and after moving to Oak Park, only Hanukkah.

We always celebrated the first night of the Jewish Passover with the traditional Seder meal and ate the unleavened crackers called

* Modern Judaism is represented by three movements: Orthodoxy, which preserves traditional practices and retains Hebrew as the language of prayer; Reformism, an attempt to retain Jewish values while adjusting practices to contemporary conditions, using mainly English; and Conservatism, which situates itself between the two. In Orthodox and Conservative Judaism, the house of prayer is called a synagogue, while reformed Jews call it a temple. On the extreme ends of the spectrum are the ultra-orthodox Hasidic communities and the ultra-modernist Reconstructionists.

matzo, even though we continued to eat regular bread as well. For the autumn festivals—the Jewish New Year and the Day of Atonement—our whole family attended the children's services at a downtown Reformed temple until my sister and I outgrew them. In those years, when Jewish populations were moving out of the city into the surrounding suburbs, membership in a synagogue or temple required substantial contributions to a building fund, and my parents were not interested in that kind of commitment.

Judaism is not only a faith, but a shared history and way of life, and my parents believed they could transmit to us, by their own example, the values they saw as being the essence of Jewish tradition. In this they were only partly successful. Their kind of Judaism was an identity, but not a personal faith, and it was never enough to satisfy my own spiritual yearning. I needed a God who was a father. I needed a God who was a saviour. I needed a God who was himself the answer to my search for meaning.

Searching

In 1960, the year John F. Kennedy became president and the year I turned thirteen, I began keeping a journal of my thoughts and inner life. I had always been conscious of the mystery at the heart of things, and my world, fed by voracious reading, was already widening. My personal spirituality contained elements of both Judaism and the Christianity I knew from books. During my third year of high school, I became friends with a classmate who was a militant atheist, and without much of an effort, I abandoned what was more a self-conscious religiosity than a deeply-rooted faith. The loss of God left an anguish in my heart, and I began searching for him anew.

I needed meaning in my life, and when I entered Michigan State University, I chose my courses and professors in the hope of finding the answers I sought. Fortunately for me, this *pot pourri* of literature, foreign languages, and social science courses filled the requirements of a humanities major.

I swung between intellectual enthusiasm, romantic entanglements, and involvement in the social movements of the 1960s. I had remained close to one of my high school English teachers, an elderly woman named Connie Young. Connie was Catholic and deeply committed to her students. Each time I returned from university on a semester break, I would go to see her, and she would listen without comment as I expounded on my latest philosophy of life. It was as if she listened me back into the mainstream of my own integrity. She never preached, never imposed her own meaning. She herself lived as if there was meaning in the universe, and she imparted to me her confidence that I, too, could discover it.

Christianity had always attracted me, and each time I entered a Catholic church, I sensed a presence I had never felt elsewhere. Between my sophomore and junior years, I spent the summer with my mother's cousin in Mexico City. Exploring the Mexican capital and environs, I found myself wandering in and out of churches, drawn by their mystery. Because it was all part of experiencing a foreign country, I didn't feel a need to analyze or justify my attraction. Life was overflowing with possibilities; I felt related to everyone and everything.

In the valley of shadows

Eleven years earlier, my father had been diagnosed with multiple sclerosis, a disease of the central nervous system for which there was no cure. As the illness progressed, he became increasingly crippled, but refused to give in to discouragement. Using electric scooters for ambulation, he continued his work in medical research.

My parents were determined to keep his condition from casting a shadow over our family life. Their intentions were well-meant, but Peggy, Mark, and I sensed the unspoken tensions without being able to identify or talk about them. It also made it more difficult for us to cope with our own feelings and conflicts about my father's illness.

During my third year of university, my brother, now thirteen, was diagnosed with bone cancer. In November 1966, his left leg was amputated at the hip. Despite chemotherapy, the disease metastasized to his lungs. He died at home, in my mother's arms, on June 22, 1967.

When we went to view Mark's body at the funeral home, I was startled by my instinctive recognition that *this was not my brother*. What had made him "Mark" had departed, leaving an empty shell. It was my first intimation of the soul.

Throughout this intense and tragic year, I had suppressed my own emotions in order to support my parents. The summer after

Mark's death, they began to surface in a confused form. My parents had learned bridge to distract themselves, and as Peggy and I sat with them, evening after evening, in the sad, empty house, I choked back the terror of becoming mired in the quicksand of my parents' grief. I had a desperate desire to break loose from the all-encompassing sorrow that clung to my family. I wanted to leave Michigan State, go to New York, and try to find myself anew, but my parents could not face another rupture in their lives. In the end, I couldn't bring myself to cause them fresh pain.

Connie Young introduced me to her spiritual director, a Detroit seminary professor and spiritual writer named Fr. Edward Farrell. It was the first time I had ever spoken with a priest, and I had no idea what I was supposed to say. Disarmed by his warmth and acceptance, I found myself pouring out my heart to him. He listened without giving advice, and my emotional turmoil began to subside.

Before I returned to university in the fall, Fr. Ed celebrated a Mass for my brother. I didn't understand all that was happening, but as he elevated the consecrated host, a ray of sunlight streaming in through the stained glass windows intersected with the paten, and the thought came to me, *this is the centre of the universe*. It was the first of many times in my life when God spoke, as it were, directly into my heart.

"To what" or "to Whom"?

Back at Michigan State for my senior year, I started attending Masses at the Newman Center and even enrolled in a Catholic Inquiry course. I was alienated, however, by the priest's presentation of St. Thomas Aquinas's proofs of the existence of God—"just in case anyone still has doubts," he said. My doubts were not allayed, and I abandoned both the classes and Mass.

During the winter semester, I signed up for a course on Shakespeare. It surprised me when my essays for the course turned out to be spiritual interpretations. I had always been uncomfortable with religious terminology that didn't seem to evoke anything with which I could identify, but when I took a course in contemporary theology and read works by Paul Tillich and Nicholas Berdyaev, such words as "creation," "sin," and "redemption" started to acquire meaning. I began to feel that faith wasn't something "out there," but something potentially within.

I still didn't know what I wanted to do with my life, but I sensed I wasn't ready to make a commitment. As my senior year drew to a close, I admitted to one of my friends, "What I'm really looking for isn't a career or a profession. I want to find the meaning of life and live it out."

After graduation, I decided to go to Boston and look for a job. Boston seemed a manageable city, less threatening than New York, and rich in history, universities, and culture. My atheistic high school friend was already living there, trying to survive as a painter, so I arranged to stay with her until I could rent a room of my own. Although I asked my parents to pay for my airplane ticket, it never occurred to me to consult them about my decision. I was finally creating my own life, but I was too insecure to do anything but plunge in blindly. I had a sense that the answers were in my heart, and I hoped that a new and unfamiliar environment might bring them forth.

After working a few months at temporary office jobs, I was hired as a social worker by the Massachusetts Public Welfare Department, my qualifications being a university diploma and a clear chest x-ray. Since I spoke Spanish, I was given a caseload of Puerto Rican and Cuban immigrants, along with a smattering of Irish-Americans.

Many families in the last group had been on welfare for generations. What could I, a twenty-two-year-old fresh out of university, teach these people about life, I asked myself. Since I couldn't pretend to be a professional, what *was* my relationship to them?

During the three-day orientation session, I became friends with a young woman named Anne, who, in the aftermath of Vatican II, had left an archdiocesan teaching order to live with five other ex-nuns in an inner city lay community. I began spending weekends with them, accompanying them to Mass, and meeting their friends. The gospel they strove to incarnate was one that made sense to me. In the absence of specialized training, Christianity (such as I was beginning to understand it) became the point of reference for my social work.

I had rejected out of hand what I saw as my supervisor's patronizing and often punitive attitude towards the welfare clients. It seemed to me that the only authentic way I could serve the families

with whom I worked was as a fellow human being, using my position and the advantages of my background to be an intermediary.
If Jesus was the Son of God, I reasoned, I truly *was* their sister. This
gave me not only the right, but also the responsibility to help them.

If Jesus was the Son of God...

There were lots of ifs. *If* there was a personal God, and *if* his essence was love, it seemed to me only logical that God would want to
express that love by sharing the condition of those whom he had created. Jesus' incarnation, virgin birth, and resurrection from the dead
were never problems for me, because *if* there was a God, he could do
anything he wished, in whatever way he desired.

I understood the Eucharist as both the agent and expression of
the fundamental unity of the human race. My Catholic friends told
me I could receive communion with them on Sundays, and the priest
didn't seem to object. It was for me a profound experience.

Boston was a hotbed of radical politics, and Anne and her friends
were becoming increasingly involved in the movement against
American military involvement in Vietnam. I was invited to a talk at
their home by a priest who belonged to the Milwaukee Fourteen, a
group of clergy and laypeople who had broken into a draft board office, stolen files, and burned them publicly to protest the war. Their
willingness to suffer prison for the sake of their convictions unfolded
for me the power of self-sacrifice. I understood it as a paradigm of
death and resurrection.

The gathering was scheduled for a Friday evening in early
March. Shortly before I left work that afternoon, a Puerto Rican
family I knew came into the office. The weather was cold and blus-
tery. They were wet and shivering and poorly dressed, with thin,
sodden shoes. They told me the heat in their apartment had been
turned off because they hadn't been able to pay their oil bill.

The Welfare Department had an established procedure for such
cases. Because it was considered inhumane to leave people without
heat and electricity, the social worker would write an order to be
phoned in to the fuel supplier so that service could be restored. I explained this to the family, adding regretfully that since it was Friday
and almost closing time, the problem would only be resolved after
the weekend.

"But we are cold," said the father plaintively.

I was genuinely sorry, but there was really nothing I could do.

I went to the gathering and listened to the priest speak about Christian protest. Afterwards there was a potluck supper. The room was stuffy, and at one point, I took off my cardigan. Suddenly I remembered my shivering Puerto Rican family.

"But we are cold!"

"I'm so sorry, but I can't do anything until Monday. I really can't."

When my brother is suffering, have I a right to say there is nothing I can do?

I told my friend Anne what had happened. She gathered up some extra blankets, and someone lent us his car. I knew where the family lived. By the time we reached their apartment, it was close to 11 P.M. The father, clad only in pyjama bottoms, opened the door; we had obviously awakened him. I could see past him into the kitchen, where the oven door was open. They had turned on the electric stove for heat, and the apartment was stifling. Feeling silly and embarrassed, I thrust the blankets into his arms, mumbled something apologetically, and retreated as quickly as possible.

But something had happened in my heart, and I never forgot it. *"When my brother is suffering…"*

Soon after this incident, I attended a talk by Fr. Daniel Berrigan, a well-known author and anti-war activist. Listening to him, I suddenly understood that there would never be social justice in the world unless those who "had" sacrificed some of what they possessed for the sake of those who "had not". The implications stretched far beyond the sphere of economics. It was what underlay the actions of the Milwaukee Fourteen as well as the sacrifices and voluntary poverty of centuries of believers. It meant that the way I lived, and the decisions I made, affected the whole world.

I had been searching for my own inner truth, but I now realized that the meaning of my life was intrinsically connected with the lives of my brothers and sisters. But that was as far as I could go. As my friends compared the merits of revolution with those of progressive social change, I listened in silence. Back in the solitude of my studio apartment, I felt ashamed of my inability to reason independently.

What came first, I asked myself, the discovery of truth or a commitment that opened the door to living in truth? To what should I commit myself? Or was the real question, to Whom?

When Welfare Rights demonstrators trooped into our office that spring, some of the demonstrators smiled and waved at me, for I was well-liked in the neighbourhood. I was disturbed, however, by the increasing polarization of positions and by the politicization of the Welfare Rights movement. After one of the leaders invited me to lunch and suggested I turn over my case files to the group, I realized it was no longer possible to remain on both sides of the fence.

I resigned my job and spent a miserable six weeks living off my savings and wondering what my next step should be.

On the Fourth of July I joined several hundred antiwar demonstrators on the Boston Common for a twenty-four hour roll call of the Vietnam War dead. When the FBI arrived with cameras and began to film the protestors, I realized the time had come to decide what I really believed in and what I really wanted to do.

I knew that Connie Young, my high school English teacher and continuing mentor, spent a part of each summer in Ontario, Canada, at a place called Madonna House. I had a vague memory of some of the things she had told me: that the community had been founded by a Russian baroness whom people called "B", and that the Baroness and her second husband, Eddie Doherty, were living as brother and sister.* Some time later, I came across Thomas Merton's *Seven Storey Mountain* and realized that the Baroness Catherine de Hueck, whom Merton had met in Harlem, was the same "B" whom Connie so admired.

Connie had spoken about the young people who were part of the community and who always struck her as being so happy. "Happy" was not an adjective I would have applied to any of my Boston contemporaries. We were searching, we were anguished, many of us were neurotic, some were on drugs, but none of us could be described as being, quite simply, "happy."

Longing to get away from the city and its intractable problems, I phoned Connie to see if I could meet her at Madonna House. She told me whom to contact. In answer to my letter of inquiry, I

---

* They had made a promise of chastity, as had the unmarried members of the community.

received a warm response from the Madonna House registrar, telling me I was welcome to come and stay as long as I wished. Enclosed with the letter was a packet of literature, the religious language of which almost made me change my mind about going. Almost—but not quite.

"You probably won't like it," Anne predicted.

My other dissident friends were even blunter. "Madonna House! They're so traditional! Why on earth would you want to go there?"

"I don't know, but I'm going," I answered with uncharacteristic tenacity.

Somewhere I had never been before

One evening in late July 1969, I boarded the Boston-Toronto bus. Sitting in the front seat, I felt that my life was about to take a decisive turn. I could see only what was immediately before me, like the stretch of highway illuminated by the bus's headlights as we sped through the night. I sensed I was interiorly heading somewhere I had never been before.

The next morning I changed buses in Toronto, and in the late afternoon, after a five-hour drive north through a country of densely forested hills and dotted with lakes, I spotted the sign for Combermere. Connie met me at the bus stop, and we drove in her car about half a mile along a winding road, bordered by pines and birches, until a large, white, two-story house came into view. Surrounding it were smaller buildings and flower gardens.

As we turned into the parking lot, Connie stopped the car to greet a man playing Frisbee, whom she introduced as Fr. B. The next person I met was called T.D.

Does everyone here go by their initials? I wondered.

T.D., otherwise known as Theresa Davis, embraced me warmly. After depositing my luggage at the dormitory for women guests, we returned to the main house to await the supper bell.

I found myself in a large, wood-paneled library-dining room with tall bookshelves set between double windows. At one end of the room stood an upright piano. A dozen or more wooden tables, flanked by benches, were set for the evening meal. The late afternoon sun streamed through the open windows, and I could smell the pine trees.

"Here comes B," Theresa exclaimed. "She knows you are here."

I turned to see a stocky woman in her early seventies advancing toward us, leaning heavily on a cane. Her silvery blond hair was piled on her head, and she wore large red earrings, bright red lipstick, and a simple blue dress reaching almost to her ankles. She stopped, looked at me, and broke into a magnetic smile. Her eyes were sapphire blue.

In a rumbling voice with a strong Russian accent, she announced, "Miriam—my mother!"

I looked around.

"She's speaking to *you*," said Theresa.

"But my name is Mary Beth," I said, confused.

"I call you 'Miriam' because that is the Hebrew name of the mother of Jesus Christ. You are named for her. You are Jewish, and your people are the ancestors of the Christians, so I can also call you 'my mother.'"

I had absolutely no idea how to respond.

"Never mind," she told me. "You don't understand yet, but you will!"

That I was Jewish seemed to mean a lot more to Catherine than it did to me. I accepted it, though—partly because I sensed it wouldn't do any good to argue, and partly because I already had the intimation that Madonna House and its Russian foundress held something for which my heart was longing.

That night I slept amazingly well for being in a dormitory with twenty-two other women. We each had a narrow bed or bunk, and only an orange crate to hold our personal belongings. I was glad I had travelled light.

The next morning, we were awakened by an alarm at 7 A.M. After Mass in the wooden chapel above the dining room, we came downstairs for a breakfast of oatmeal, homemade bread, butter, and jam, and steaming hot tea. It was so delicious that I hardly noticed the absence of coffee. Along with other guests, I was then driven in a van up a country road, given a container to tie around my waist, and turned loose on a hill laden with raspberries sparkling like jewels in the sunlight. Compared to the inner and outer confusion I had left behind in Boston, this was a pastoral idyll.

The following day, another girl and I were assigned to shovel compost onto flower beds near the main house. Laying aside my responsibilities for war, poverty, and interracial justice, and abandoning my veneer of sophistication, I found myself laughing at the sheer incongruity of the situation. It came to me with a start that I was—happy!

At first I was puzzled that no one asked me where I was from or what I had been doing. Even when I offered the information myself, no one seemed particularly interested. Someone eventually explained to me that personal questions were discouraged out of sensitivity to individual situations. This rationale became more understandable when a fellow guest told me confidentially that she had been sent to Combermere by her parole officer.

The absence of identifying information made conversation difficult at first, but as I and the other guests became immersed in Madonna House life with its all-embracing spiritual focus, and as we were drawn further into our own inner journeys, we found ourselves relating to each other naturally and at a depth we could not have anticipated.

As my Boston friends had predicted, I found the Roman Catholicity* of Madonna House foreign in many aspects. One evening before supper, as I entered the little chapel above the dining room, expecting to pray vespers as we normally did, someone handed me a rosary. My reaction was visceral and atavistic; suddenly and without warning, I had become a lone Jew in an alien, Gentile world. Sliding in along one of the wooden benches, I fell to my knees and prayed desperately, "God, if you exist, you have to do something!"

Each decade of the rosary was prayed in a different language. Catherine prayed in Russian; someone else—in French. Then a priest began to recite, "*Avinu, she ba-shamayim*...Our Father, who art in heaven..."

---

* I didn't have the spiritual background to recognize the Eastern Christian accents that were such a distinctive feature of Madonna House spirituality. Catherine Doherty was teaching the community to breathe from what John Paul II would later describe as the two lungs of the Church, its Latin and Byzantine heritages.

I had never studied Hebrew. I didn't understand the words, but the sounds evoked memories of the children's services at Temple Beth El on the Day of Atonement and of my father's humorous attempts to resurrect his Bar Mitzvah Hebrew at our family Passover celebrations. The language was part of my past, and, it would seem, my present. It was as if the Mother of God was trying to reach me in an idiom permeated with associations, the language of my personal history and communal identity, the language of my heart. This was what Catherine had been trying to convey to me at our first meeting, and I recognized it as the answer to my frantic prayer.

Despite such "anachronistic" elements as rosaries, and even the life-sized bronze statue of Our Lady of Combermere, I found at Madonna House none of the oppression and puritanism my Boston friends and I had attributed to the institutional Church. On the contrary, I was overwhelmed by an atmosphere of gentleness and joy and by the acceptance of each person as he or she was. The words *Pax-Caritas*, Latin for "Peace and Love," engraved on the silver cross worn by community members, expressed a tangible reality. In contrast to the world I had just left, there was a marked absence of aggression and competitiveness, of manipulation, and of sarcastic or demeaning humour. Instead there were frequent peals of wholehearted, childlike laughter. As I joined in, I felt like a young plant unfurling its leaves in warm, spring air.

Wasn't the Madonna House life an image of the kind of world my friends and I were dreaming of? Where did it come from? How did they do it? My friends and I were seeking to dismantle an unjust, exploitative society, but what were we going to replace it with? Were not the roots of the very ills we deplored to be found in our own hearts?

Shyly, awkwardly, I tried to articulate my questions to Fr. Brière, the Frisbee-playing priest who had become my spiritual director.* His answers were simple and to the point. My intellectual facade notwithstanding, it was by intuition—a quality I hadn't even known I possessed—that I grasped what he was saying: that the problems of society were the result of original sin, and the answer was always

---

* Each Madonna House guest was offered the possibility of individual guidance from one of the priests belonging to the community.

Jesus—turning to him, recognizing our sins in the light of his love, confessing and being forgiven, being healed, receiving and sharing his love. I didn't have to be afraid of my weakness. On the contrary, it was the inability to acknowledge my need that kept Jesus from pouring into my heart the power of love, which was another name for grace.

The ease with which I found myself moving in this new reality frightened me. I sensed Jesus saying to me, *"I am the Way, the Truth and the Life,"* and I longed to reply, "My Lord and my God." But every spontaneous movement towards faith was sabotaged by self-analysis. Trained in the tenets of the sociology of knowledge, I knew that what people accept as truth is highly influenced by the social environment in which they find themselves. What appeared to me as the growing credibility of Christian doctrine might only be the effect of the love and acceptance I was receiving at Madonna House. It would be many years before I would come to understand that spiritual truth cannot be evaluated by psychological, sociological, or political analysis. Faith is a response to a different reality.

God calls me Miriam

I had only planned to stay at Madonna House for a week, but I found myself swept from one day to the next, caught up in the momentum of my pilgrimage. Madonna House's hospitality was such that "working guests," as we were called, could remain up to a year without a commitment. Six weeks after my arrival, I told Catherine I would like to go back to Boston to sublet my apartment and then return to Combermere for an indefinite stay.

"Wouldn't it be better for you to go learn what it means to be Jewish?" she asked.

I heard myself say, "I think it's too late for that."

She fixed on me her penetrating, blue-eyed gaze for what seemed an eternity. "So. You have met Jesus Christ."

I felt she was looking into my heart and seeing there more than I recognized myself.

"Very well. Come back and stay for awhile. But it won't be as you expect."

I didn't understand what she meant by "it won't be as you expect," but I have always been grateful for her suggestion that I leave to become "more Jewish." Not only was it something I could use to counter my family's suspicions that I was being proselytized, but it also increased my own respect for Catherine and my trust in her. *

When I phoned my parents in Oak Park to let them know of my plans, they couldn't begin to picture the place I was trying so inadequately to describe.

"It's like a Christian kibbutz," I said finally.

My father asked flippantly, "Oh, are you going to become Christian?"

"I don't know. Not yet."

There was dead silence at the other end of the wire.

"We'll talk about it when I come home," I said quickly, sensing my mistake.

Only afterward did I realize how devastating those few little words had been for my parents. The death of my brother had left a gaping wound in their lives, and they were painfully vulnerable. They themselves hadn't realized how much Judaism meant to them until I casually, without any forethought, put into the air a possibility that would sever (at least from their point of view) one of the deepest threads of continuity left in their lives.

Several months later, after I had returned to Madonna House from Boston, my mother wrote me a long letter:

> I can see in retrospect that I was not right in thinking I could flaunt the customary ways of instilling in you an appreciation and acceptance of Judaism. Without the reinforcement of Jewish education, life holds too many obstructions, too many difficulties and forces to contend with. I wanted you and Peggy to have a love of our heritage, an appreciation of its ethics and morality, without the ritual and all that to me seemed without meaning. But this isn't possible—or if it is, it needed a better teacher than I. I wasn't experienced or knowledgeable enough to bypass what I disliked in the hope

---

* Anti-Semitism is widespread in Russia, and Catherine's esteem for Jews was atypical. Her father, Theodore Kolyschkine, had learned from the great religious philosopher Vladimir Soloviev to love and honour the people who had given Christ to the world, and to help them in times of persecution. Catherine had been taught to do the same.

of giving my children the essence of what Judaism is to me. It wasn't fair to you children not to have given you a way of life and a purpose.

We wanted to live in an area with enough of a Jewish population to protect you from the feeling of being completely different, which was so much a part of my own life. We wanted to give you a sense of identity and to spare you the anti-Semitism you were already beginning to sense around you.

As you have said, there is bigotry and prejudice in Catholicism and in all religions; in Judaism too. But the precepts of love, compassion, and humanity, which you are seeing in the people you admire and respect, are also found in all peoples, not only in the Catholic Church

You say that you are not rejecting your Jewishness, but I cannot see any compromise between Judaism and Catholicism. The fundamental tenet of Judaism is, "Hear, O Israel, the Lord our God, the Lord is one God." *One*, Mary Beth, only one. If you believe in God, there is only one God, not three.

Personally, I don't believe in a God, whatever one's interpretation is. And Judaism is the only faith where you can reject God and still have enough left to live honestly. What is Judaism? It is a faith, and if you take that away, it is a culture, and if you deny that, there is a sense of history, of tradition, and above all, a moral and ethical code that all men can live by. I think it's nice to believe in God—it gives you something to hang on to in times of trouble, though I can't use that kind of a crutch myself. But whatever I profess to believe or not believe, I am still a Jew in my own eyes and in the eyes of the world.

Love alone is not the answer. Love is a means to accomplish aims beyond our own selfish desires. Love for others is the instigator of effective action. But don't make the mistake of thinking love is the solution—it isn't. Love in its highest form was the way I felt about my husband and children and their potential for themselves and for humanity. I thought it was a shield that could keep out all that was evil. But all the

love in the world, and all the prayers it generated in people
of all faiths, couldn't save Mark. Mark died, and I knew
there was no God. Love wasn't enough.

Love is a lot, but it isn't enough. It is a means to go on
living for the sake of others, but it isn't going to solve everything for you or me or anyone. Whatever is to be accom-
plished has to be done on more honest, realistic terms.

You have used the word "love" so often in your letters
and when we have talked that I am sure it is the basis for
your thinking, but your father and I cannot accept "love,"
whatever your interpretation or application of it, as a reason
for turning from Judaism to Catholicism. Our love for you
and Peggy has been so immense that it transcended our own
needs and wishes, in the midst of great grief and loneliness,
to give you both the freedom to live your own lives. You cannot ask us now, in the name of love, to give our blessing and
understanding to the denial of our heritage and yours.

When I finished reading the letter, I fled to the chapel and wept
silently for a long, long time. Madonna House people were not
afraid of tears, and they seemed to have a way of discerning when
people needed space and when they needed a compassionate presence. Presently, I felt a hand on my shoulder. I looked up to see Jean
Fox, one of the staff workers.

I told her briefly what my mother had written.

"Be at peace, sweetheart," she said. "You follow God, and he will
take care of your parents. You'll see."

I wanted desperately to believe her.

As shaken as I was by my mother's pain, I did not let her argu-
ments sway me. An instinct I could not identify helped me stand my
ground. I would later come to understand this instinct as the presence of the Holy Spirit in my heart.

Meanwhile, I had my own questions about the Church and its
teachings—especially those related to marriage and sexuality. Fr.
Brière broke through my resistance with an inspired explanation.

On a piece of paper he sketched a wheel. "Here, at the hub, is
the Holy Trinity—Father, Son, and Holy Spirit," he told me, pointing

with his pencil. "This is where you always have to begin. All the is-
sues you are concerned about are like points on the rim. If you start
there, you will go around and around in circles. But if you start at
the centre, with the Trinity, you can follow the spokes to any point,
and you'll understand the real meaning."

I was almost ready to ask for baptism, but I still agonized over
one fundamental question: did God really exist, or was I was creating him from my own need? This was the dilemma on which everything else hung. I could not resolve it intellectually, and it came to me
that the only way out of the impasse was to take a step in faith.

New liturgical rubrics had just come into Church practice, and
over a period of six weeks, in the presence of the whole community,
I went through the stages of Christian initiation. Fr. B. had decided
against a formal catechesis. Participation in the rich spiritual life of the
community had augmented the background I had acquired through
reading, even before coming to Madonna House. Perhaps he felt I
needed the sacramental graces more than intellectual preparation.

Several days before my baptism, Catherine came over to me at
afternoon tea.

"Well, Mary Beth," she began, "now that you are going to be
baptized, I had better get used to using your baptismal name!"

I had become so accustomed to hearing her call me Miriam that
my original name sounded strange on her lips. The thought passed
through my mind: *God calls me Miriam!*

On the last Sunday in Advent, December 21, 1969, I was baptized Miriam Elizabeth in the Madonna House chapel. Connie Young
and Fr. Edward Farrell drove up from Detroit to be my godparents.
I felt little during the actual baptism. The heavens did not break
open, and I did not have a revelation of Jesus. Still, for several weeks
afterwards, I found myself wrapped in a wordless sense of God's
presence.

Upon his return to Detroit, Fr. Farrell went to see my parents and
broke the news to them. Though he phoned me the next day to say
the meeting had gone well, I suspected that my parents simply would
not permit themselves to pour out their heartbreak to someone they
hardly knew.

Eventually my mother wrote:

No matter what, I do not want to lose you because of my feelings and needs. I will keep on struggling to maintain what I most deeply believe—the right of every human being to seek the meaning of life as he or she sees it.

If I regress sometimes, please be patient, and know that I will fight my way back. Sometimes I have to resort to defences to shield myself from the hurt until I learn to cope with it. I don't know if the hurt is for you or for me, or for both of us.

I can't understand, but I will try to accept. And I love you.

She added in a postscript that my father had not been able to put his feelings into words, but had cried after Fr. Ed's visit. I wrote to him that only because of the love he had shown me all my life could I believe in the existence of a loving God.

Where I am able to hear him

Anyone who spends a protracted length of time at Madonna House usually finds himself asking, "Could this be my vocation?" As I continued to share the life of the Madonna House family, as I was touched and transformed by the love I received, I began to wonder what could be more meaningful than to dedicate my own life to loving in this way, to becoming an apostle of love. Had I not longed to find the meaning of life and live it out?

The community's simple lifestyle, with its emphasis on the kind of manual work most middle-class North Americans were endeavouring to escape, struck me as an identification with most of humanity and, consequently, as an affirmation of the dignity of every human being. I was awed at the depth and breath of Catherine's vision. It began with the spiritual restoration of the individual, and as each person learned to make his or her life a work of love, he then became a leaven for social change and the restoration of all facets of human life. "Nothing is foreign to the Apostolate," Catherine loved to repeat, "nothing except sin."

On the other hand, I had never even remotely considered the possibility of taking vows* of poverty, chastity, and obedience. The promise of chastity was the most confronting. Before coming to Combermere, I had been seriously in love several times but had not been ready to make a lifetime commitment. I had always assumed that someday I would get married.

Now, while I continued to long for human intimacy, I was becoming aware that a kind of existential solitude, in which I always found my deepest reality, had been present in my life from childhood. This was the source of the authenticity Connie Young had recognized and affirmed in me. When I could stand apart from the opinions and expectations of those around me, I rediscovered my own being. Loneliness led me to what T.S. Eliot called the "still point in the turning universe," the profoundest experience of my own truth. The bridge between this "being-in-solitude" and the yearned-for union with others was Christ.

Fr. Brière articulated it much more simply: "Give your heart for others, but keep your heart for Christ."

Neither Fr. B., Catherine, nor anyone else in the community tried to influence me. After celebrating my first Easter, I left Madonna House to try my wings as a Christian "in the world." I went to Quebec City and found work at a YWCA cafeteria. I was delighted at the opportunity to apply the principles I'd learned at Madonna House, but became over-involved with the directress of the "Y", who turned out to be an alcoholic. Shocked at the discovery, wanting to help but without any understanding of the illness, I badly mishandled the situation. When the directress was fired, I lost my own job as well. Emotionally battered and with my self confidence shaken, I returned to Madonna House to sort things out and to discern my next step.

This second stay was much more difficult. I found the community and its way of life much less attractive on a natural level, but I couldn't make a clean decision to either leave or stay. When he thought I had flailed around long enough, Fr. Brière sent me off to one of the little cabins set aside for twenty-four hours of prayer and

---

* Called "promises" in Madonna House. There is a canonical distinction, but the essence is the same.

fasting. He instructed me to take a sheet of paper, draw up two columns, "Reasons for Going" and "Reasons for Staying," and jot down everything that came to me without analyzing or editing it.

I followed his instructions:

Reasons for Going

• I am afraid to stay.

• I am afraid of the consequences of poverty, both physical and intellectual.

• I don't know if I am suited for community living. I need both privacy and free time to find my centre.

• I am afraid of losing touch with the reality other people live in. I have found comfort in living the questions and am afraid of having the answers.

• I don't understand celibacy. "Giving my heart to Christ" seems an abstraction.

• To "leave father and mother" in my case is a very radical and even cruel step.

• Do I even have real faith?

Reasons for Staying

• I am afraid to leave!

• I am afraid I will not be able to live as a Christian in the world. Without the support I find here, I'm afraid I will get distracted and succumb to illusions.

• I'm afraid I am too weak intellectually, emotionally, and spiritually to survive elsewhere.

• I am tired of the same stops and starts. I am afraid that my weakness will forever keep me a dilettante at life. If I settle down with a commitment, I can start to grow up.

• The purity of this life appeals to my search for something absolute.

• When I think of living Christianity seriously, I see the need for poverty and self-renunciation. Because of the forces in society and my own susceptibility to self-indulgence, I need to do this in a radical way.

• *I cannot live without God. Here, he is the centre of our life. I am able to hear him.*

If this is the deepest meaning of my life, I thought, why on earth would I want to risk losing it? What was I trying to prove?

I left the cabin and went joyfully to inform Fr. Brière that I most probably had a vocation to Madonna House.

Your People Will Be My People

Soon after my first promises, I went to spend the first week of my holidays at our field house near Washington D.C. I was to spend the second week in Oak Park with my parents, and the prospect had me swimming in anxiety.

I tried to hide it. In fact, I tried not to feel it. I had just finished a very intense year of being trained in community living, and I wanted to enjoy this time of leisure and freedom. But even as I struggled to project the image of being at ease in my role as a new staff worker relaxing on holiday, I could feel my *persona* disintegrating and my hidden terror beginning to surface.

I had always known I was impressionable and that I tended to take my sense of identity from those around me. I felt like a patch-work quilt composed of bits and pieces of those I admired, and now the fabric was falling apart. What if my decision to become a Catholic and to join Madonna House were only reflections of a need to be accepted, a need to belong? I didn't dare let the question form in my conscious mind.

One night, as I lay in bed, I felt myself falling into a bottomless black well. As I tumbled into its depths, a mocking voice screamed over and over, "You are no one! *No one*! You have no identity!

"You are nothing!

"*Nothing*!

"*NOTHING*!"

The echoes became a roar as I fell, faster and faster, into a pit of darkness.

Just before the final annihilation, I had a sense of being caught and held in loving hands. Into my heart came the words, *I live; not I, but Christ lives in me* (cf. Gal 2:20).

This was who I most essentially was, the identity no one would ever be able to take from me. This was the reality I had not been able to fully comprehend at the time of my baptism.

Awaking the next morning, in the moment between sleep and full consciousness, I felt as if I were standing on a pearly white beach, washed smooth by the waves, under a sky streaked with rose and gold.

It was not that simple

Catherine had never wanted me to lose my Jewish identity, but I knew I first needed to acquire one. In the years that followed, I read everything I could find on Judaism. I read novels by Chaim Potok and Elie Wiesel. I read Max Dimont's *Jews, God and History* and Abba Eban's *This is My People*. I read Abraham Heschel, Martin Buber, and Franz Rosenzweig's *Star of Redemption*, in which he attempted to reconcile Judaism and Christianity. Later I began to study Hebrew and learned enough to decipher my grandfather's prayer book and the first chapter of Genesis. A chill ran up my spine as I read, *"Bereshit barah Elohim et ha-shamayim v'et ha-arets";* "In the beginning, God created heaven and earth." Not only was Hebrew "my" language, it was the language of God himself!

Equally adamant that I claim my heritage was Lebanese-born, Melkite-rite Archbishop Joseph Raya, whom I had first met in Combermere in November 1969. Ten years earlier, he had been serving at a Byzantine Catholic parish in New Jersey when friends brought him to Combermere. Madonna House had an immediate impact on him as "a place where East and West live together in love and harmony." He became the first associate priest of the community, part of the spiritual family, while continuing to serve in his own parish. On August 15, 1969, shortly after becoming archbishop of "Haifa, Nazareth, Akko, and all Galilee" in Israel, he ordained Catherine's husband, Eddie Doherty, a priest in the Melkite rite.

Even at the time of our first meeting, I was Jewish enough to feel a personal relationship with Israel and to be excited that he had come to Madonna House from "my" country. I was also painfully aware of the injustices experienced by Arab Christians in Israel, and I found myself saying to him, "I am so ashamed of what my people are doing to your people."

"Sweetheart," he answered, "you and I know that this is a family affair. But when Christians love and forgive, we show to the world the face of Our Lord Jesus Christ. If we do this, he will be visible, and the Jews will recognize him too. This is our task!"

"Be sure you stay Jewish," he told me.

For Catherine and Archbishop Raya, as for most Christians, salvation history was an unbroken continuum from the Old Testament to the New. From this vantage point, however, what did one make of the two millennia of rich Jewish life and developing thought *after* Christ's death and resurrection? For Christians, acceptance of Jesus of Nazareth as the Son of God is the fulfillment of Judaism, but for Jews, it is the ultimate rupture after which one no longer belongs to the Jewish community. I knew from the beginning that if I "became more Jewish," as I was so consistently being urged to do, it would bring me to a new confrontation. When I reached that crossroad, who would be able to help me?

My first mission assignment was in Winslow, Arizona, where we lived in a predominantly Mexican-American community. I loved the Hispanic culture and the closeness to the people, who gave us their hearts without reservation. After four years in this little "room of Madonna House," I was transferred to what we called a "poustinia-prayer house" in Gravelbourg, Saskatchewan.

A decade earlier, Catherine had introduced the Russian word *poustinia*, meaning "desert," into the Madonna House vocabulary and life. Drawing on Russian Orthodox tradition, she set aside small cabins in Combermere, and rooms in our various field houses, where staff workers and visitors could spend twenty-four hours at a time in silence and solitude, fasting on bread and tea, meeting God in the Scriptures and in their hearts. With the publication of the book *Poustinia: Eastern Spirituality for Western Man* and its subsequent translation into many languages, the concept became known throughout the Catholic world.

The Gravelbourg foundation was the third MH poustinia house. Instead of active apostolic work, its mandate was one of prayer and listening—listening to those who came to our door, and listening to God as he spoke in our hearts, in our guests, and in our lives. For Catherine, prayer encompassed everything one did and was. Every service rendered, every activity performed with love, was prayer. Striving to live before the face of God and to serve him in one's brother, a person "became a prayer." The poustinia was not only a room where each of us spent twenty-four hours each week; it was a life that made no sense without God and that taught us to stand in the desert of our hearts where we could be led by the Spirit to the living springs of divine life.

I had barely begun this journey when my mother was diagnosed with a rapidly spreading cancer. I returned home to be with her and my father during the last few months of her life. The Nazareth life of simple everyday service that I'd learned in Madonna House gave me the tools to care for her lovingly and peacefully, to stand with her in faith, and to support my father and sister. Shortly after my mother's death in August 1977, we discovered that my father himself was terminally ill with an advanced stomach cancer. He died six weeks later.

During my five-month stay in Oak Park, I found myself immersed once more in the world where I'd grown up. As an adolescent, I'd chafed at its narrowness; now I was fascinated by the rich ethnicity. After my father's death, while my sister and I were arranging to sell our family home, I took advantage of the opportunity to attend synagogue services, enrol in night courses, and take part in the Saturday morning Torah discussion group at a Reformed temple. I continued to go to Mass at a nearby parish and participated in a Catholic charismatic prayer group. This busy religious schedule was a buffer against the loss I was not yet ready to confront directly.

My sister and I agreed that I would sort through and organize my parents' papers and possessions. Together we would decide what to give away or sell, and she would take care of the final clearing out. The work went smoothly and peacefully, and by the end of November, I was free to resume my own life. I returned to Combermere for a rest, and after New Year's, I went back to Gravelbourg.

At the crossroads

I knew I had to let myself grieve. Each week I would go into poustinia and sob until I had no more tears. Then I would write whatever came into my heart, letting the words spill onto the pages of my journal without editing or analysis.

January 6, 1978

I know I have to live in the present, but I am tormented by questions that prevent me from letting go of the past. The self who left Gravelbourg last spring, who survived all those months by clinging to God, and who was strong in him seems to have vanished into thin air.

In Oak Park, I was surprised to find a new grounding in Judaism. I thought I had left that world, but in my time of need, my roots called out to me, and the aloneness was alleviated.

Back in Combermere, I was consoled by the love of the Madonna House family, by Catherine's compassion and respect for what I had lived. Here in Gravelbourg, I have re-entered a traditionally Catholic world, and I suddenly feel like a stranger.

What happened? What have these eight years since my baptism been about? Did I don a new set of clothes and call it conversion? Is that all my Christianity consisted of?

There is deep, deep truth in Judaism. Its history is the history of man, in his weakness and his grandeur. It has searing questions—how to live in a world created by God, but seemingly abandoned by him; how to live in waiting and in hope; and how to guard the flame amidst the forces of destruction. There is heroism and nobility and poignancy.

Is Jesus the answer to these questions?

I don't really know Judaism, and I am beginning to think that I don't know Jesus either.

All this time, I clung to faith in the one God—*"Hear, O Israel, the Lord your God is the one God."* (Dt 6:4) I was no longer sure of anything else. I grieved for my parents—not for their deaths, but for the suffering that had filled their lives and which seemed to have defeated them in their final years. I could not touch the reality of the resurrection and refused to cheapen it by painting pictures of paradise in my imagination. All I could do was to face the silence head-on, letting the pain of standing naked before God smash against me like breakers on a storm-swept beach. I tried to stand still in the void and begged God to show me reality.

January 26, 1978

I am realizing to what an extent my decision to become Catholic and to join Madonna House was an act of rebellion against my parents. It was as if I had been trying to shield my life from their unhappiness. While this was not my only motive, it was stronger than I ever wanted to recognize.

Now they are gone. They were the memory of my past, and I am left in a room with only three walls, open to the storm winds.

On some level, the call of Christ and the truths I recognized still hold. *"You have not chosen me: I have chosen you."* Before, it never seemed difficult to leave father, mother, brother, sister, land, and people. The difference now is that I have come to love them.

In his biography, *The Pillar of Fire,* the Jewish Christian psychiatrist Karl Stern quotes another writer as saying that when a Jew dies to rise with Christ, the whole people must die with him. He is right. Caiphas tried to prevent it: *"It is better that one man die and not the entire nation."* It is because *"in Christ, there is neither Jew nor Greek"* that Jews have fought conversion so fiercely.

I cannot celebrate both the Jewish Sabbath and the Christian Resurrection. I cannot live in two worlds or pretend they are the same.

To walk in faith, to *"stand still and know that I am God,"* to remember God's acts in the past and let them be a guarantee for the future. This is the Judaism I am called to live.

February 3, 1978

Archbishop Raya was here for five days. The morning he left, I went to his room and talked with him as he packed. He himself doesn't see any difficulty in being both Jewish and Christian, but he acknowledges that from my standpoint, the situation could be problematic. His view has always been that Jesus completed the Law by bringing freedom to the individual. He sees the Jewish mind as the mind of Christ and considers the loss of this attitude to be a loss to Christianity.

He said that when Jews wanting to be baptized came to him in Galilee, he always advised them to go back and live as "real Jews"—as believers in Christ, but remaining Jews, in a Jewish community. I asked him if this was to avoid accusations of proselytism, but he said it was because of the divisions that otherwise ensued.

This I have experienced. For a Jew to become Christian brings not peace but a sword.

Over and over, the archbishop emphasized that no one can tell me what is right. I know that. I have to find the truth in my own heart, before God. I have to find the direction of the deepest current within me.

Jesus, help me not to accept the easy answers, but to let you forge your answer in me.

In December I will be taking my final promises. The idea of not having children is so alien to Judaism that a commitment to chastity *forever* is, in itself, an implicit severance.

February 11, 1978

JoAnne and Patti* said to me yesterday, "You don't have to hang on to being Jewish—you *are* Jewish!"

Their comment alerts me to the danger that what began as an authentic search could easily become another attempt to create an identity for myself. I had thought I was beyond this, but I seem to be teetering on the brink of a familiar trap.

February 24, 1978

In poustinia today I asked God why I could not simply live in the full, rich, loving way I had come to associate with the essence of Judaism. In my heart I heard:

It is too late. That was what I wanted at the beginning. But the world I created was invaded by sin, and now it is filled with forces of destruction set loose by the wrong choices. That was why I sent my Son and why you must cling to him for your life. That is why you must give him your life.

Could this be my answer?

Opening the Scriptures, I read, *"When the Spirit of truth comes, he will lead you to the complete truth, since he will not be speaking as from himself but will say only what he has learnt."* (Jn 16:13)

---

* Staff workers at Madonna House in Gravelbourg

"I have told you this, so that you may find peace in me. In the world you will have trouble. But be brave: I have conquered the world." (Jn 16:33)

March 10, 1978

I cannot live two lives, and Madonna House and Christianity are the deepest reality of my heart. It doesn't all fit together easily, but I have the sense that God is in the space between what I know and what I don't know.

Over and over, I keep making the decision to live here and now. Jesus is saying to *this* young woman, *"Your only real choice is between yourself and your neighbour."*

I am reading Martin Buber on Hasidic Judaism and am finding in it great light and peace. It seems to me he comes close to the essence of religious Judaism and to religious living when he says that the task of man is to hallow the world by the way he lives. This is also what Catherine is saying.

March 23, 1978 – Tuesday of Holy Week

Was the Passion really the way it is described in the Gospels? I know how stories become distorted in the course of history, yet the Passion has been taken literally for two thousand years. The Jew in me cringes—how many times have Christians left their churches on Good Friday and poured into the ghettos to avenge the death of Christ? If God inspired the Scriptures, as we believe, how could he have permitted the errors of history to result in so much evil in his name?

Never before have I asked these questions.

This year I stand at the edge of the crowd, having believed in this Man and no longer understanding anything.

Lord, I wish I could just throw myself at your feet in love and faith and surrender. I have to do it another way. Please understand.

April 7, 1978

So many memories have surfaced now. How little I understood what my mother went through after Mark's death! Truly, she was a great woman. She had many faults, much wounding, but she loved. She went as far as anyone can go without faith. She and my father were unsung heroes, each in different ways, struggling with life in its beauty and its tragedies. How painful that it has taken their deaths to bind me to them so deeply!

In Jewish tradition, we live on in the hearts of others and in the life of our people. But what does this really mean? Lives go on—they have to.

Lord, help me to believe my parents are with you. Show me what this means.

April 15, 1978

Between the words I speak and the heaviness I feel stands a gaping chasm, but truth is greater than my feelings. Feelings are neither right nor wrong; they just "are." I accept them, but I cannot base my life on them. I stand instead on the knowledge of what God has done in my life, on the authenticity of those moments when the Spirit has spoken in my heart. On the knowledge, to which I fight my way again and again, that he alone has words of truth and life. And I stand in the present.

May 2, 1978

As we prayed Vespers last Sunday, I cried out silently from the depths of doubt, impotence, and grief, *Lord, what is it that you want of me?*

I want you to surrender. Just put yourself in my hands. Trust me.

His words are more real than my own emotional turbulence, deeper than grief, deeper than my questions. Like Job, I have been touched by the living God.

May 27, 1978

Over and over again, I return to my original call, which I paraphrase in this way: *"There is only one thing you have to do: find a place where you can hear me speak. To do so may not be easy in our world, but this is the choice you must make if you want me in your life. You can't have it both ways, Miriam. You end up running in too many directions. If you want me in your life, find a place where you can hear me, and then stay there and listen."*

He doesn't answer my questions or allay my doubts or accede to my demands. He says, *"Trust me."*

My conversion to Christianity was not from Judaism, but from secular humanism. Now that I have begun to recognize in Judaism my deepest roots, how do I claim this tradition while remaining true to what God has been saying to me these past nine years? The answers, I think, are to be found in the experience of my weakness, selfishness, and need of a saviour.

In a broken world, Judaism is also in need of salvation.

The wound of my parents' deaths could not be transformed into some easy image of an afterlife. I am just now beginning to have a sense that all is not ended for them; that despite the pain and suffering that filled their lives and overwhelmed them in their last years, they were not ultimately defeated. Their courage and love and real goodness have an enduring significance. This, for now, is my intimation of resurrection.

In the psalms and in all Jewish experience, the living memory of God's work in the past becomes the ground for present faith. It isn't a question of going *back* to Judaism, but of moving forward in the present moment, in the continuing mystery, with God.

July 16, 1978

Into my mind the other night came the image of my mother. It wasn't a dream, not even an experience. The image took form in my consciousness, and I let my imagination build on it. The picture was very clear and very tender. My mother was well, her face freed of the tension of illness. Her voice was full of love and concern as she told me not to mourn for her and my father.

"Honey, you don't have to worry about us. We want you to live your own life."

I know this was what she had always wanted for my sister and me. It was part of her greatness, the way she tried to live. At times she succumbed to her own weakness and needs, as we all do, but this was the real foundation of her love.

It was as if she were telling me to let go of my father and her, telling me that I must not build my life on their illnesses and deaths, but on the truths I have experienced. This is what they would have desired.

"Leave father, mother, brother and sister, and come, follow me." (Cf. Mt 19: 21, 29)

August 18, 1978

Next week it will be a year since my mother's death. Jewish tradition prescribes eleven months of mourning. I sought neither to mourn nor to let go of mourning, yet both seem to have happened naturally.

I have learned much this year. Inherent in my new consciousness of family and community, and in my ties to Jewish history, has been God's desire that I give it all back to him. For a long time I was not able to face this. Now, very gently, I let it go, not watering down the tensions or seeking to resolve them, but following the living God, day by day.

France

After two more years in Gravelbourg, I was transferred to Madonna House Ottawa in the fall of 1980. The following spring Catherine announced the opening of a new mission in Avignon, in the south of France. Theresa Davis (the "T.D." who had greeted me when I first arrived in Combermere) was there already, and Réjeanne George and I were to join her.

Several months earlier Catherine had met the newly-appointed Jewish Christian archbishop of Paris, Jean-Marie Lustiger. Some time before that, she had had a dream about a Jewish bishop, and when she visited Lustiger in Paris, "their souls met," as Fr. Brière later described it. She understood Lustiger's suffering over the controversy aroused by his nomination. "For me," he said in an interview, "[it]

was as if, all of a sudden, the crucifix began to wear a yellow star."[*]
He begged her to pray for him and for his priests.

Archbishop Lustiger's appointment to Paris and his connection
with Madonna House through Catherine were signs to me that my
assignment to France had significance far beyond my dream of living
in Europe. I felt a deep bond with him and a personal call to carry
him in prayer.

One night before I left Combermere, I was unable to sleep and
sat reading in a corner of the dorm where there was a night-light.
Jean Fox stumbled past on her way to the bathroom, turned back,
and stood over me, rubbing her eyes.

"You're ready, Miriam," she said. "You've come through something in Gravelbourg and Ottawa, and you are ready to go. Be at
peace. You've been faithful to what God has asked. You go and support that bishop. Support him in your heart, by your love, and in
your prayers. You don't have to be near him. Just stay faithful and
be at peace."

From the day that Réjeanne and I arrived in Paris, without the
slightest effort or initiative on my part, I found myself bumping into
Jewish Christians and Christians interested in the Jewish roots of
Christianity. The scars of the Holocaust were still raw in Europe,
and in the survivors I met, the fear of a new persecution was always
just beneath the surface. For the first time, I realized how protected I
had been as an American Jew.

Before leaving for Avignon, Réjeanne and I were invited to a private Mass with Archbishop Lustiger at his residence. I could hardly
contain my anticipation as we made our way on foot across the city.
Never before had I encountered a Jewish Christian as secure in his
identity as Jean-Marie Lustiger. I knew from his statements at the
time of his appointment to the see of Paris that he saw his baptism as
a completion, not a renunciation, of his Judaism.

Arriving at the archbishopric, we were asked to wait while the
archbishop finished talking with journalists. When he finally joined
us, Lustiger greeted us warmly, recalled his meeting with Catherine,

---

[*] During the Second World War, all Jews in Nazi-occupied countries were ordered
to wear a six-pointed yellow cloth star sewn on the left breast of their outer clothing,
identifying the wearer as a Jew. Failure to comply was punished by immediate arrest
and deportation to a concentration camp.

and apologized that we would have to begin Mass immediately, since he had another engagement afterwards.

That night I wrote in my journal:

> I am sure he realized I was Jewish, but the meeting was in the context of what had *already* taken place. Our relationship as Jews is now expressed through the Christian faith of which he is an apostolic witness.
>
> As the Jewish archbishop raised the consecrated species and prayed, "Through him, with him, and in him," I suddenly knew that the unity with the House of Israel for which I so intensely longed, the true oneness to which Judaism witnesses, is most perfectly realized in Eucharistic communion—in Jesus Christ.
>
> I was overwhelmed with joy and thanksgiving.
>
> It is written in the Talmud that whatever happens to one Jew happens to all Israel. The integration taking place in my heart has repercussions far beyond me. This is my vocation as a Jewish Christian.

In Avignon, I came to know Fr. Jean-Miguel Garrigues, a Spanish-born theologian interested in the relationship of Judaism and Christianity. I learned much from him. His beautiful exegesis of chapters nine through eleven in St. Paul's Epistle to the Romans was a healing balm on my heart. In these chapters, he explained, there is not an "old Israel" and a "new Israel," but "one Israel of God,"

In another Scripture class, this time on the sacrifice of Isaac, he pointed out that genealogical descent in the Bible is not merely biological—the "children of the Promise" were all born to sterile women. I remembered with a jolt that my maternal grandmother had been divorced by her first husband because of her supposed sterility. One could say that I, by extension, was also a child of the Promise.

Fr. Jean-Miguel placed the sacrifice of Isaac in the context of the spiritual journey from faith in God's promises to faith in the Author of the Promise. Faced with a divine command that seemed to negate the promise of "descendants as numerous as the grains of sand on the seashore" (Gen 22:17), Abraham seemed to have only two choices. He could ignore the command on the basis that God could not possibly be demanding such a terrible and incomprehensible action, or he could assent fatalistically, denying, in a sense, God's very nature. He did neither. He obeyed, never ceasing to believe that God was a God of goodness and mercy, and that from this unfathomable sacrifice, the Lord would bring life.

I wrote:

> This was also Job's answer. It was the answer of those Jews who marched to their death in the Nazi concentration camps singing, "*Ani ma'amin*...I believe in the coming of the Messiah, and even if he tarry, yet will I believe."
>
> The agonizing question, "How can one continue to believe in a God of mercy and goodness after the Holocaust?" finds its answer in the response, "Not to believe is to give Hitler a *spiritual* victory."
>
> Elie Wiesel* holds that the Jewish position is never to choose between God and his creation. In one of Wiesel's plays,** Abraham, faced with God's incomprehensible silence, leaves paradise to join the victims on their way to the gas chamber. It is then, moved by this act of love, that God begins to weep.
>
> The love we bear our brother *is* God's love. It seems to me that the essential link is always the sacrifice of one's own life for the other.

"He is risen!"

In January 1983, after reading about a Carmelite monastery that had been founded just outside the gates of the former concentration camp at Dachau, Germany, the idea of making a pilgrimage to the camp began to take root in my heart. I wrote to the Carmelite sisters, asking if I could stay with them for a few days during Lent.

This would be a pilgrimage to the very heart of the Jewish wound. I wondered if something within me would be integrated. I wondered if I would be torn apart.

---

* Survivor of the Bergen-Belsen concentration camp and author of many novels and plays with the Holocaust as their theme.
** As this play is not listed among Wiesel's works, it must have been written by another author. I've never been able to find it again!

Marie-Thérèse Huguet, a friend of Fr. Jean-Miguel's from Paris, was spending the night with us, and when I spoke to her of my idea, she offered to arrange with friends in Munich for me stay with them on my way to and from the nearby concentration camp. Since the Carmel at Dachau had not responded to my letter, I decided to telephone them. If they accepted me, I would take it as a sign I was really meant to go.

Their answer was affirmative. The prioress later told me that even had there been no room in the guest house, knowing I was from Madonna House, and that I was Jewish, they would have taken me into the cloister.

On the train to Germany, I began reading a talk Cardinal Lustiger had given to a Catholic gathering in Düsseldorf the previous year. As a boy, he had spent the summers of 1938 and 1939 with a German family in Munich, and he described in the article the emotional turmoil he experienced when he returned to Germany for the first time after World War II. To forgive, he explained, does not mean to forget, because we cannot pretend that what happened did not take place. True pardon does not deny death, but transforms it. Pardon is the victory of Jesus crucified and risen, but still bearing his wounds. These wounds, however, are now transfigured; they have been transformed into signs of healing and salvation. When we allow our hearts to be converted, we unite ourselves with God and share in the pardon founded on the victory of Christ, the victory that transforms death into life.

As these thoughts found a place in my heart, the knots in my stomach began to loosen. God is in this land also, I thought as we sped across Germany. I was not travelling into death, but into a deeper knowledge of God's mercy and forgiveness.

The previous year, in the spring of 1982, I had attended an international charismatic gathering in Strasbourg, on the Franco-German border. I remembered my reaction to the presence of thousands of Germans at the conference—that instinctive stiffening, the questions and accusations I'd been surprised to discover in my heart. Where were you *then*? What did you know? What was your involvement? God's word to me at that time had been unequivocal: I too must forgive; I too must let down my historical defences; I too must let my wounds be healed. Perhaps now—after the Israeli-Lebanese war of the summer of '82, the horror of the refugee camp massacres, and my own confusion as I tried to sort it all out—I understood better that wounds aren't eradicated as if by a magic wand. They must be touched by grace in order to become one with the wounds of Christ and, in him, sources of healing and reconciliation. Only when we cling to God, in a conversion that surrenders to him our past, present, and future, does true healing take place.

At the Munich train station, I was met by my host, Albert Kurlanczek. We drove to his home, where I met his wife, Elisabeth, and their five lively children. Elisabeth was Catholic and a member of the French charismatic community Emmanuel. Albert was a Jew from Avignon. He was stunned that I, an American Jew, baptized Catholic, living in his native city, would come voluntarily to Dachau to touch the cataclysm from which I personally had been spared.

It was my turn to be stunned when Elisabeth mentioned that her prayer group had been praying for me—even before she had received my letter—at the request of a recently baptized Austrian Jew who had heard about me through Marie-Thérèse Huguet, the same person who had put me in touch with the Kurlanczek family!

That afternoon I joined Elisabeth and her friends on their weekly prayer walk at Dachau. Moving slowly through the camp, we prayed the rosary before the Catholic memorial, the Jewish memorial, and the plaque dedicated to the Poles who had been martyred at Dachau. The prayer was simple and unpretentious, and I was touched by the sincerity, although the bright charismatic songs seemed inappropriate to the sober setting. We concluded with a time of adoration in the Carmelite monastery chapel, just past the gates at the end of the main camp road. As I said good-bye to the prayer group, I felt the strength of their love and support. I no longer felt alone on my pilgrimage, and I had a growing realization that I had not come for myself alone.

Dachau, the first concentration camp established by the Nazis, had been used as a model for the camps that followed. Not only Jews had been imprisoned there, but also thousands of Germans, Poles, and other nationalities, including more than 2500 priests. To me, the presence of the Church in the hell of Dachau was a witness of Christ's identification with all victims.

The sky was overcast and grey as I walked through the camp the next day. The silence chilled me to the bone. Everything was neat, everything was silent, everything was empty. The original barracks had been razed; two had been reconstructed. In the museum were photographs, descriptions, history, items belonging to prisoners.

The crematorium was spotless, surrounded by cypress trees. I tried in vain to remember the Kaddish, the Hebrew prayer for the dead, and instead I found myself praying, over and over, "Jesus Christ, Son of the Living God, have mercy on me, a sinner." It was as if that Name alone had power over the evil that had reigned here.

I stood at the edge of the silent ash grave, before the remains of thirty-six thousand lives. "Thirty-six thousand" seemed more personal, somehow, than six million. Thirty-six thousand individual existences, individual destinies, living, breathing, laughing, loving, and now reduced to one six-by-two foot grassy knoll.

I tried to take it in.

In the silence of Dachau, I heard the angel's voice.

"Why do you look for the living among the dead? He is not here. He is risen."

At Mass that evening in the Carmelite cloister, I received communion and stood for a long moment, gazing at the host in my hand. My whole being trembled. To receive the Body of Christ was to receive *all* those for whom he died. It meant communion with the executioners and communion with the victims.

"In Christ, there is neither Greek nor Jew," and I, too, am a sinner in need of God's mercy.

Raia and Volodya

THE RUSSIAN CONNECTION

Catherine could never explain why she closed the house in Avignon two-and-a-half years after its foundation. The tensions in Europe, with the Soviet Union and NATO both installing nuclear missiles on their respective sides of the German-Czech border, were not the real reason; she was responding to a deeper intuition she could not articulate.

I didn't understand, and I was devastated. I loved the house, loved our life in Avignon, and loved being in Europe. I felt as if I were presiding over the demise of my own child.

"Remember, Miriam, not the promise, but the God of the promise," Fr. Jean-Miguel reminded me. His words came back to me one luminous evening in Combermere in 1985, when it was announced that Cardinal Lustiger had invited Madonna House to open a prayer-listening apostolate in Paris. We had been offered two apartments in a church rectory in one of the oldest districts of the city, and Réjeanne George and I were to be the first team.

From our first days in Paris, we felt that the spirituality of the poustinia was what Madonna House was meant to offer in France. People continually expressed their delight at finding a place of solitude and prayer hidden in the heart of the city. Our three poustinia rooms were often full, and those who came appreciated our availability and hospitality.

As usual in Madonna House, there were changes in personnel. Ill health necessitated Réjeanne's return to Combermere in 1988, and I was named director. In the summer of 1991, the staff worker who had been with me for several years was reassigned to another mission, and Teresa Reilander was appointed to replace her

While awaiting Teresa's arrival, I decided to do a thorough cleaning of our apartments. From morning until evening, stopping only for Mass and to grab something to eat, I scrubbed, sorted, culled, and gave away or jettisoned everything we didn't need or use. The house was quiet. No one was scheduled for a poustinia that week; there were few calls and almost no visitors. It was gratifying to do physical work and even more gratifying to have a sense of renewed order in the house.

I was perched on the kitchen counter, scrubbing down the walls. Above me, the paint was several shades darker, but the ceiling was so high I would have needed a taller ladder to reach the upper part of the wall. Someday we would have to repaint the whole room, I thought, but the project called for someone with greater skill than I had.

The phone rang. Lowering myself gingerly from the counter, I went to pick up the receiver. A deep male voice said in slightly accented English, "My name is Vladimir. I am Russian. Someone in Taizé told us about you, and my wife and I would like to come visit."

"That would be wonderful," I responded, calculating rapidly in my mind. Today was Tuesday; in a few days, the cleaning would be finished…"Why don't you come for supper on Friday?"

I barely registered the brief silence at the other end. "Very well. We will come on Friday." I gave him directions and hung up.

Accustomed as I was used to the Parisians, who planned their schedules well in advance, I hadn't thought twice about putting off the visit until later in the week. I didn't know that in Russia, it was customary to say, "Come right over!" or at the very latest, "Come tomorrow!" Nor could I have known that Vladimir Erokhin and his wife, Raia, had just arrived from Taizé, an ecumenical community in eastern France that receives thousands of young people each year, and were phoning from the train station. All they knew about us was that we were a community in Paris, founded by a Russian. They were under the impression we were a women's monastery, and monasteries usually had guest houses.

Unaware of having committed a cultural gaffe, I happily completed my housework and prepared for my guests a meal combining Parisian presentation with Madonna House simplicity. I made a soup of blended leftovers, a salad, and even bought a few different kinds of cheese, which I arranged on a platter. Dessert would consist of pastries donated by the St. Vincent de Paul group that met at the rectory on Wednesdays. I brought out a bottle of red wine in honour of the occasion.

Raia and Volodya, as I learned to call him,* were an attractive couple in their mid-forties, about my own age. They later told me how surprised they were to see a woman in high heels and earrings running down the stairs to greet them. Clearly, this was not an Orthodox monastery!

My lovely meal never got the attention it deserved. There was so much to share that we hardly noticed the food. In fact, it was with difficulty that we broke off conversation so I could clear the dishes for the different courses.

Volodya, who spoke fluent English, translated rapidly for his wife. The couple lived in Moscow; Raia had a grown daughter by a previous marriage, who lived in Israel. Raia was delighted to learn that I, like her, was Jewish. Volodya's father had been a Communist. Volodya himself was a journalist and musician, Raia was an artist, and they had a small Christian publishing house and theatre group.

Both were spiritual children of Fr. Alexander Men, an extraordinary Orthodox priest of Jewish background, whose brutal murder the previous fall had been widely reported in the French Catholic press. The Erokhins' lives bore the imprint of Fr. Alexander's vibrant faith.

I told them about our community, Catherine's life, the poustinia, and our apostolate in Paris. Although Volodya was translating everything from English to Russian, on a deeper level it was almost as if I was speaking a language they already knew. We all felt it.

God had brought these Russians into the Madonna House orbit. Where would it lead?

In the weeks that followed, our friendship deepened. Raia made a poustinia, and they returned many times to talk about their life and about the problems and decisions they faced. There was an extraordinary sense of communication, but when I heard Raia complain to her husband, "I wish I could talk to Miriam by myself," I was moved to buy a beginner's Russian textbook to see what I could pick up. When I shyly mentioned this to the Erokhins, I was surprised at how touched and encouraging they were.

They told me that their apartment in Moscow was always filled with friends and members of their theatre group, and that Raia, in

---

* Most Russian first names have diminutives, which are used by family and friends, e.g., Vladimir–Volodya, Raissa–Raia, Tatiana–Tanya, etc.

particular, was exhausted from the constant comings and goings. I was glad we could offer them the silence and peace that were so intrinsic to our house.

As a rule, we tried not to mix the different guests who came to see us, since most people had personal concerns and had not come to socialize with each other. One Saturday afternoon, however, turned into a three-ring circus. The Erokhins arrived as scheduled, but were barely inside when someone else knocked at the kitchen door. Mercifully, Teresa Reilander had arrived from Canada the week before and took the new arrival into the living room while I visited with our Russians in the kitchen. Fifteen minutes later, two more friends arrived, one of them a Russian-born Jewish Christian from Israel! Soon she and the Erokhins were deep in animated conversation.

When Teresa and I were alone once more with Raia and Volodya, I apologized for the hubbub. "Your lives are so busy, and you are both so tired, that I wanted this to be a place where your hearts can rest," I told them. "I didn't want to shut you up in the kitchen!"

"But it was wonderful!" they protested.

"In Russia, the kitchen is the centre of our life," explained Volodya. "That's where we bring our close friends. Russian lives are always full of people and noise. This is how we live. It just makes us feel more relaxed with you."

Our kitchen had a counter along two walls, instead of a table, and uncomfortable barroom stools. It certainly wasn't homey in my estimation, but I was glad he liked it.

The Erokhins were struggling to discern the next step in their lives. Raia was afraid of the mounting anti-Semitism in Russia and wanted the security of an Israeli passport. The rest of her family was already living in Israel, and her daughter was begging Raia to come. Were the couple to apply for immigration, they would be given assistance by the Jewish Agency, but Volodya, an ethnic Russian, doubted that he could live outside his own culture.

The situation seemed complicated, and we, having been well trained in discretion, didn't ask a lot of questions. It looked as if they might have to move in separate directions, at least temporarily. Their French visas had already expired, and if Volodya intended to return to Moscow, he would have to leave as soon as possible. In order for Raia to go to Israel, however, she would need to spend another couple weeks in Paris completing the necessary paperwork. In view of her language limitations, neither Teresa nor I could envision her staying alone.

One of the cardinal rules of the Paris apostolate had always been that, except for poustiniks, we could not offer overnight accommodation to anyone except visiting Madonna House staff. Réjeanne had impressed this on me from the outset in order to safeguard the spirit of our poustinia life—it was all too easy to get distracted.

In this instance, however, Teresa and I thought God might be calling us to make an exception. Not only was Raia comfortable with us, but the bond we were developing with her and Volodya had deeper implications, which I couldn't yet articulate. I knew it had to do with Catherine. After checking with Jean Fox, who was now Director of Women,* we invited Raia to stay with us when Volodya left and until we ourselves went on holidays in early August. The Erokhins were both moved by the offer.

And so, one Saturday afternoon in mid-July, Teresa and Raia accompanied Volodya to the Gare du Nord. Among the three of them they carried: a Russian typewriter, a clarinet, a violin, a synthesizer, a music stand, and one small case of clothing. After Volodya's train had chugged out of the station, Teresa and Raia returned to Madonna House, where, during the next ten days, our friendship continued to deepen.

We communicated in pidgin English and Russian, with constant referrals to a dictionary. Most of all, we used our hearts. As we could only get across the essentials, we found ourselves becoming simple and childlike.

That Raia was an actress was definitely to our advantage. She had us in stitches as she mimed scenes from her visits to the Jewish Agency, where one official had taken a most unprofessional interest in her. Another evening, a French friend joined us for dinner, bringing an assortment of cheeses. We explained the different varieties to Raia: "Baa-aa-aaa" for sheep's milk, "moo-oo" for cow's milk, and a nasal "aa-aa-aaa" for goat cheese. When we heard ourselves, four

---

* Catherine died on December 14, 1985. Shortly afterward, Jean Fox was elected Director General of Women and served in that capacity for three-and-a-half terms until her death in 2004.

adults in their thirties and forties, cavorting with animal noises, we collapsed in laughter.

Of course, there were things we didn't understand and inevitable cultural blunders. Raia spent a few days at the country home of one of our friends and returned with a bag of clothes she had been given and which she wanted to share with us.

"*Podarki*–gifts!" she exclaimed happily.

"Oh, no, they are for you," we insisted. Using the dictionary, I tried to explain that we had a promise of poverty and tried not to keep items we didn't need. Raia didn't understand. When I saw the joy leave her face, I realized my mistake. She was the recipient of our hospitality, and now she too wanted to give. I tried to make amends, but the damage was done.

I learned from that incident, however, and when she wanted to help out in the house, I was alert enough to accept the offer. Observing the speed and efficiency with which she peeled and sliced vegetables and then whipped through a stack of ironing, Teresa and I quickly revised our preconceptions. This woman might not speak a foreign language, but in her own milieu, she was obviously anything but helpless!

I took her through the Rue des Rosiers, the old Jewish quarter of Paris, a few blocks from our house, but she didn't respond as I had expected. "I am Jewish, but my soul is Russian," she told me. I later came to understand that she was typical of her generation. Just as Russians in general had lost a sense of their spiritual heritage, most Russian Jews, while retaining their ethnic identity, knew little about Judaism as a faith.

On the day of her departure, I accompanied Raia to the Orly airport, from which she was to fly to Tel Aviv. It was mid-August, and the place was jammed. Raia stuck close to me, saying over and over, "I'm so glad you are here!" After we had registered her bags, a female Israeli airline agent approached her for routine questioning.

"Are you her interpreter?" she asked me. I nodded. "Ask her whether she packed her bags herself or if anyone helped her."

I turned to Raia. "You—suitcase," I began in pidgin Russian. I made a packing motion, pointed to myself, then shook my head and made a face.

Raia easily understood what I meant, but the agent, seeing I was not the translator I claimed to be, hauled Raia off to a professional. By the time she returned, we just had a few minutes for a cup of coffee before her flight was announced.

It was hard to say good-bye.

With Jean's encouragement, I continued to study Russian throughout the fall and winter. I couldn't believe how hard it was, but the language acted on me like a narcotic. I couldn't get enough of it.

Raia wrote from Israel and again after her return to Moscow in January. When I spoke to them by phone, Volodya reiterated their invitation to visit.

At the Directors' Meetings in May, I asked Jean for permission to spend my summer holidays with the Erokhins in Moscow. The trip would be a pilgrimage to the roots of Madonna House, to Catherine's roots. Although a friend who had traveled several times to Moscow was dubious about the advisability of going by train, I decided, after praying about it, that I would either take the train or not go at all. I wanted to get the feel of the land, the continent of Europe, the spaces of Russia. I also had a sense that this would be a journey into poverty, perhaps my own.

Jean gave me her blessing.

"THIS IS RUSSIA!"

Monday, August 3, 1992 – Train from Paris

Teresa accompanies me to the Gare du Nord. My luggage consists of my own suitcase, a second large suitcase with gifts and supplies for the Erokhins, and a bag with food for the train. A young woman approaches me on the quay and asks me to take a package to Moscow, where her mother will meet me at the train station. As items are regularly stolen in the mail, and this seems to be the customary way of getting packages to people, I accept.

The train pulls out from the station—and I am on my way to Moscow!

My three-bunk compartment is not uncomfortable. I will have it to myself until we reach Warsaw tomorrow afternoon. In the car there is a congenial atmosphere. Next door are two nineteen-year-olds—Hélène is French, Katia has been visiting her in Paris, and now they are travelling to Moscow, where Hélène will spend time with Katia's family. It seems as if most of the French people in the car have already been to Russia. The two car attendants speak only Russian.

Tuesday, August 4, 1992 – Train

What a pleasant surprise to be asked this morning by one of the attendants if I would like some tea. They serve it in glasses with little silver holders like the ones we have in Combermere.

In Warsaw, we have an hour's wait. On the quay are stands where food and drink are sold, and since I have no Polish currency, I ask a vendor in Russian if she will take either dollars or francs. She says no, because she doesn't know the exchange rates. When I press her, she opens a bottle of lemonade and pushes it toward me, indicating she doesn't want any money. I wonder if it is because of my Madonna House cross.

The quay is packed with Russians laden with bulging bags, knapsacks, and worn luggage. Katia says they come to Warsaw in order to buy merchandise to sell back in Russia. The new capitalism. She doesn't seem to like it.

Our car has filled up. I am now sharing the compartment with Vika (short for Viktoria), who looks to be in her early thirties, and her eight-year-old daughter, Marina. Vika is a doctor. We share food, and she insists on buying me tea. Tomorrow, when we say good-bye, I will give her the rest of my sausage, which she likes, and some little perfume samples I brought along as gifts.

Just past the border between Poland and Belarus, there is a three-hour layover in Minsk while they change the wheels on the train, since Russian railroad tracks have a wider gauge. Katia has realized that the arrival times given us in Paris were based on Parisian, not Moscow, time. She wants to phone her family and offers to call Raia and Volodya for me. To say this is not as simple as it sounds is an understatement. The first challenge is to find a phone that works. Next, to keep getting telephone tokens from a surly attendant, who seems to think there should be a quota per customer. I try my luck with her and am successful—foreigners always receive better treatment, Katia informs me. Since the phone connection only lasts thirty seconds, it takes her five tries to shout the arrival information to her family. She manages to connect with Raia on only the second try.

We wait a couple hours on the platform, watching for our train to reappear. Katia is trying to hide her nervousness that we might not be at the right place. The station is shabby but clean, and thronged with people and baggage. Old women are pushing heavy mops. The people from our car gradually come together, and when the train pulls in, we race to find our car. When we left Paris, only two of the cars were destined for Moscow, but in Warsaw, Moscow-bound cars from all over Europe were hooked together, and the train is now very long. I now understand why Volodya asked me on the phone for the number of our car.

Wednesday, August 5, 1992 – Arrival in Moscow

When I awake this morning, we are in Russia! Or maybe it is still Belarus; no one seems to know for certain. It doesn't matter. I spend all day standing in the corridor, gazing out the window. Birches... pine...wooden houses.... The countryside has a different quality to it. It's not gentle or rolling as in France; not picturesque as in Germany. There is nothing cozy about this country. It is simply—endless. All day I see only one or two churches. Before the Revolution, they must have stood in the centre of every village.

By two-thirty, we are travelling through the suburbs of Moscow, and suddenly, we are in the station! How am I going to get my luggage out of the train? I wait for most of the passengers to get off, but then, to my horror, new ones are already boarding! Suddenly, to my joy and relief, there is Volodya at the door of the compartment.

Quickly, he takes the situation in hand. There is no question of my carrying anything. Slinging my heavy suitcases over his shoulder, he grips my hand luggage with one hand and me with the other and manoeuvres us out onto the platform. The woman whose daughter had entrusted me with the package is waiting. I hand it over; she thanks me and is gone. I dare not look around for fear of losing Volodya in the crowd. We push our way down into the metro. People, people, people everywhere! Built by slave labour during the 1930s, the Moscow metros are ornate, with chandeliers hanging from the ceilings and mosaics on the walls. In contrast to the Paris metro, they are also spic and span. It is hard to talk over the noise of the train, so Volodya and I just smile at each other.

The Erokhins live on the second floor of a five-storey brick apartment building in northeast Moscow. Inside their apartment, the walls of the entrance hall are covered with posters from theatrical productions, some of them their own. There is a good-sized kitchen, a small bathroom with a sink, tub, and semi-automatic washing machine, a toilet cubicle, and two bedrooms. In the larger room are bookcases reaching to the ceiling, a sofa-bed, a large wooden desk, several chairs piled high with books and papers, a baby-grand piano, a large electric synthesizer, and various other musical instruments. The walls are hung with original paintings. The second room, where I am to stay, used to belong to Raia's daughter, Yana. Crowding the shelves and decorating the walls are homemade theatrical props: masks, a sceptre, crowns, and even a miniature throne. Everywhere there are books, photographs, paintings, and a sense of warm, rich cultural life.

Into this apartment flows a constant stream of people. Some belong to the Erokhins' wide circle of friends, others are part of the theatre group, and still others are involved with the forthcoming bus trip to Taizé.

We gather in the kitchen, and I remember what Volodya told me in Paris about the kitchen being the centre of Russian life. They have just repainted it in honour of my visit. I can see where the paint, a pale yellow, ran thin toward the end, but they tell me proudly that the room looks much brighter now. Potted plants line the windowsill and the tops of the wooden cupboards painted by Raia in Russian designs.

When they ask if I am hungry, I start to say no, thinking 5 P.M. must be too early for supper. Then I realize the question is rhetorical—any time is mealtime in Russia, and this is the moment for a welcome celebration! We sit down to potatoes served with oil, brown bread, cheese, tomatoes, and cucumbers with fresh dill and chervil. Afterwards Raia serves fruit and cookies, along with tea made from a very strong essence and diluted in the cup with boiling water.

We converse in Russian! I manage to express the thoughts I've been rehearsing all month and make a good guess at the Erokhins' responses.

In the evening I accompany them to a school gymnasium for a meeting of the theatre group that, in two weeks, will be travelling to Taizé and Germany to present a Passion play staged by Raia. I plan to return to France with them on their chartered bus. When we arrive, about forty people are gathered, sitting on mats on the floor. They have brought an icon and a candle. We pray Orthodox prayers, read from the Gospels, sing Orthodox hymns and Taizé refrains. I can hardly believe it is all happening. Nor can I believe it when Volodya introduces me and asks me to speak about Madonna House—in Russian! I make a valiant start and then, realizing how ridiculous it is—after all, I've only been in Moscow three hours!—ask Volodya to translate. After speaking briefly about Catherine, I am able to add in Russian, with all my heart, "I'm so happy to be here with you!"

Thursday, August 6, 1992

Coming into the kitchen on my first morning in Moscow, I confidently greet Volodya with the Russian words, "*Good evening!*" He doesn't bat an eyelash and answers politely, "Good morning, Miriam."

Raia and I go walking downtown. What strikes me, as we make our way to Red Square, is the disordered profusion of small vendors selling every imaginable item at unimaginable prices. It is capitalism Russian style, a whole new way of life that seems to have sprung up almost overnight.

There is nothing oppressive about the city, even in Red Square. The queue waiting in front of the Mausoleum to file past Lenin's embalmed body consists primarily of foreign tourists. Raia says quietly, "Only when Lenin's body has been buried will Russia be free."

I didn't expect to have a spiritual experience on my first day in Moscow, and I certainly didn't expect it to happen right on Red Square, in St. Basil's Cathedral. The latter is a fantastic whirl of colourful, twisting towers. Built not for public worship, but for the Imperial family, it has a central iconostasis, the sides of which wing out at angles to form multiple chapels.

The cathedral is being renovated. It is full of cement dust and building supplies, but as we wander through, I find myself suddenly riveted before an older iconostasis. For the first time in my life, I

understand what is meant by the "presence" of icons. Our Lord and
Our Lady are tangibly before me. I begin to weep. In this church,
which was turned into a museum for seventy years, on a square that
was synonymous with Soviet power, not only is God present, but he
has always been present! He has never left, has never abandoned
this country. The church may have been made into a museum, but
the presence of God in these icons transformed the museum back
into a church. Man cannot kill God. Man cannot abolish God. Such
is the power of his resurrection.

Was this what Catherine was always trying to tell us? Was this
why she reacted so angrily to suggestions about "converting" Russia?
I want to cry out, "Now I understand! God is here; he is and was
and always will be!"

Since I need to change money, we make our way to one of the
big hotels for foreigners. At the entrance, Raia asks a uniformed
guard where we should go, and in reply, she receives a blank stare.
I try my luck as a foreigner and am given polite information, which
I pretend to understand. When we approach the proper entrance,
another guard refuses to let us pass. Then Raia does something that,
she later tells me, was for her highly uncharacteristic. She looks at
the guard straight in the eyes. As if her lack of fear pierces his veneer
of power, he lets us through.

I change twenty American dollars. The exchange rate being one
hundred and seventy roubles to the dollar, I now have the equivalent
of Volodya's monthly salary. I feel as if the money is burning a hole
in my billfold. My mind can't encompass the disparity.

We have been invited to dinner at the apartment of Volodya's
sister, Olya. Her husband, a psychologist, is away at a meeting in
Riga. Also present are Olya's nine-year-old daughter Katia, a young
American Protestant missionary who is finishing up a stay in Moscow,
and an enchanting little woman of indeterminate age called Sonia.
The meal is simple: rice, bread, cheese, cucumbers, and tomatoes.
We sit on a rickety sofa and a motley collection of stools, crowded
around a small table in the cluttered kitchen. I don't understand
most of the rapid conversation, but am content simply to be present,
enjoying the warmth of being together. I already feel as if I've been
a year in Russia!

By the time we return home, it is 11 P.M., and the phone is ringing. For the next two hours, Raia takes one call after another. She is the main organizer for the forthcoming trip, and there are endless problems and complications. She explains to me, "Nothing is easy in Russia. Now you see why we are all so worn down."

Friday, August 7, 1992

We leave the apartment early to catch the train to Tver, three hours away, where we will spend the weekend with Volodya's mother, Lilia Stepanovna.* This is an opportunity for me to see the countryside and an ancient Russian city, once a centre of culture and where the old wooden houses have been preserved. In the rush to get off, they forget the food they are bringing, and Volodya has to go back for it and catch a later train. His sister and niece join us at the station. In the crowded car, we stand for the first hour. Raia is exhausted; it's good for her to get away from the phone and the worry. We talk about Judaism and Judeo-Christianity. Olya, who speaks excellent English, is quite interested. Among the French charismatic groups in Moscow is the community of the Beatitudes, which integrates some of the Jewish traditions and is present in their Orthodox parish.

Tver is a typical provincial city, and the slower pace is a relief after the crowds and bustle of Moscow. I thought I wasn't allowed to travel more than forty-five kilometres outside the capital without official permission, but I'm told that no one cares any more. My visa also says I'm supposed to register within twenty-four hours of my arrival, but they all laugh and tell me not to worry about it. They explain that neither before nor after the Revolution have Russians paid much attention to laws. People learn to get around anything they can.

Lilia Stepanovna is a simple, fast-talking woman of sixty-six, with henna-dyed hair, who used to nights in a bread factory. Now retired, she still works a night shift as a watchman at the archives building next to her apartment house. I learn that Volodya's family is from the Tambov region, where Catherine's parents had their estate. By

---

* The polite way to address an older person or a person with whom one is not on casual terms is to use the first name followed by the patronymic, generally with the ending –*ovitch* for a man and –*ovna* for a woman.

the time Lilia Stepanovna was born in 1926, the Kolyschkines had been long gone, and the name doesn't mean anything to her.

Lunch is a typically Russian meal with cabbage, tomato, and egg salads, *pirogi*, *blini*, and marinated fish. In France, there is only one dish for each of the prescribed courses, but here there is a profusion of dishes, a sense of largess and freedom that I find refreshing. They serve a special vodka that everyone downs with one swallow. Among the different sweets is a concoction of pure sugar that you put in your mouth and through which you suck your tea—always, there is tea. They bring out a silver samovar and set it on a tray. This is a modern samovar that heats the water electrically. Perched on top to keep hot is a smaller teapot containing the strong tea essence.

Raia and I go for a walk, leaving Volodya, Olya, and Katia to bathe in the Volga River, which runs through the town. We talk and talk. Despite my limited vocabulary, Raia and I always understand each other. Back home, Lilia Stepanovna has left for work. There is another meal, after which Raia takes a nap, and the rest of us go walking again.

Olya tells me about her conversion fifteen years ago, when she was twenty-three. She had seen an icon print and had sensed the reality behind it. Then she read the Bible. Volodya, who had been baptized six months earlier, brought her to Fr. Alexander Men. Olya described how Fr. Alexander had instructed them: groups of students would arrive by train from Moscow after nightfall. One by one—in twos at the most—so as not to arouse the suspicions of the villagers, they would slip quietly through the side door of the church. On weekends they would come from the city to sing in the choir. The day Fr. Men was murdered, it was as if their own lives had ended. Olya and her husband had collected the dirt that was soaked with his blood.

She told me how she would go to the Tretyakov Gallery with her drawing pad to secretly pray before the icon of Our Lady of Vladimir. Each time a school group came through on tour, she would step back and pretend she was sketching the icon. Many Christians did this. One day she was astounded to see someone furtively kiss the image of Our Lady. Today, in the new Tretyakov Gallery, the icon is behind glass for protection, but in front of it always stands a vase with fresh flowers.

It is a relief to be able to speak English with Olya and Volodya. With the exception of Raia, who speaks to me slowly and distinctly, I've been disappointed at how little I can comprehend. Lilia Stepanovna's rapid-fire conversation is almost completely unintelligible. To compensate, however, I seem to be drawing on an intuitive capacity I never knew I possessed.

Back at Lilia Stepanovna's, we drink still more tea and sit around talking about art and theatre. This time, I can follow the gist of the conversation, and now and then, they translate. The play they will be presenting in Taizé and Germany depicts the Passion of Christ. Is it good, they ask, for a person to play Judas or the devil? Is there not a danger that we become what we represent? What do I think? I say that we are not simply at the mercy of random spiritual forces. If we are living Christian lives and receiving the sacraments, we are protected by the power of Jesus and by the faith of the Church. They like that, but there is still speculation about the spiritual vulnerability of the artist. I enjoy the relaxed atmosphere and the conversation of people who are comfortable together.

Saturday, August 8, 1992 – Tver

The heat and mosquitoes make it an uncomfortable night for everyone. I was given Lilia Stepanovna's bed since she was working; tonight they will set up a cot for me in her room. The others are sleeping on mattresses on the dining room floor.

Raia is relaxed just being away from Moscow. We go shopping, and I realize why it is that Russian streets look so different from city streets in the West —it is the virtual absence of display windows exhibiting merchandise. Everywhere there are kiosks selling a variety of Western goods, but the prices are prohibitive. In government-run stores, prices are lower, but also the quality, and the selection is limited. These stores look like empty warehouses with counters hugging the walls, each selling a different category of food: meat and fish (very expensive), dairy products and eggs (hard cheese is expensive, but we buy a lot of *tvorog*, a drained cottage cheese), bread, and canned goods. There is also a counter where clothing is sold. You tell the salesperson what you want, she tells you the price, you wait in a queue to pay the cashier, and then go back and wait again with your ticket to collect your purchase.

We spend the day walking in old Tver. As I didn't bring a camera, I try to fix the scenes in my heart. These one-storey painted wooden houses with carved window frames must be like those of Catherine's era. They have no indoor plumbing and are heated by coal or wood stoves. Old Tver had somehow escaped destruction by the Communists, though parts of the city had been heavily bombed during the Second World War.

We walk in shifting pairs. Volodya tells me about the struggles of the past year and his need to find God again. We compare our student days in the sixties. Like my friends and me, Volodya and his friends had rejected the power of the industrial-military complex. No one believed the official anti-American propaganda; on the contrary, they were fascinated by the United States and curious about the reality of American life. Volodya says perestroika was a direct result of Reagan's Star Wars program, because the KGB realized they couldn't compete with the U.S. militarily and sought another kind of change.

On a country bridge overlooking a little stream and waterfall, Olya and Volodya muse about the way language reflects the contradictions in their society. The Soviets did away with traditional conventions of social address, such as *gospodin,* "sir," and *baryshnya,* "young lady," replacing them with *tovarisch,* "comrade," and the harsh *grazhdanin,* "citizen." Today these terms have been banished from the vocabulary, and when, on a bus, someone had jokingly called me *tovarisch,* the other passengers told him angrily not to use that word. But when I asked Volodya and his sister what to say instead, they shrugged helplessly. "We say, 'young man,' 'girl,' 'woman,' 'grandmother.' It's as if we are reverting to the biological reality. We've lost the sense of etiquette; we don't even know how to relate to each other."

Olya tells me about some of the extraordinary old women she knows, who paid for their convictions with labour camp sentences. She speaks of Fr. Alexander Men's family. His Jewish grandmother was healed by St. John of Kronstadt, who said to her, "You are not baptized, but I see in your eyes that you know God." Fr. Alexander's mother was secretly instructed by an underground priest who lived in hiding for twenty years in a house in Zagorsk. "These are our treasures," says Olya simply.

I buy flowers for Lilia Stepanovna—I'm getting used to the custom of gift giving! I've already given her chocolate and a scarf I brought from Paris and have received, in return, a macramé hanging she made herself and a set of postcards of Tver.

After supper, Olya asks her brother to work with Katia, who is learning the violin. I shyly suggest we have a musical evening. Olya and Volodya both sing, and I have spotted a guitar in the corner. It is missing a string, but Volodya tunes it anyway and begins to play songs he composed twelve years earlier, before meeting Raia, when he and Olya were traveling across Russia. Despite an initial enthusiasm, the evening somehow falls flat. Everyone seems sad, but I don't understand what is really going on. Later, Raia tries to explain. "It was from another time, another Russia, another era in our lives. All that is gone now."

Sunday, August 9 – Tver

I had taken it for granted that we would all go to church today, but it didn't happen. I'm not sure why. Was it because none of them are at home in traditional Orthodoxy? Or out of consideration for Lilia Stepanovna? Olya had told me that when her mother learned of her children's baptisms, she burst into tears and cried, "I have no children any more!" Volodya said his father just considered it one of Volodya's many eccentricities, but since Pyotr Erokhin was a party member, it was important that the baptisms remained secret,

"My father was an honest Communist," Volodya explained. "He really believed in Marxism. We lived in different worlds, and there could never be any dialogue."

After her husband's death, Lilia Stepanovna gradually softened. Olya now brings her Fr. Men's books and the New Testament, but she doesn't know if her mother reads them.

We take a three-hour walk in "a real Russian woods," gathering wild raspberries and strawberries. They teach me the name of the beloved rowanberry tree, *pyabina*, which is found throughout Russia. When I tell Raia how Catherine used to say that Russians are either children of the woods, the river, or the steppe, Raia exclaims immediately, "Then I am a child of the woods!"

Raia's childhood was happy and free, but her adult life has been full of hardship. Her daughter by her first marriage became deaf

at the age of two when a physician prescribed too strong a dose
of antibiotics. Raia brought her to Moscow for special schooling.
Her husband, an artist, could not get permission to work in the
capital. Their relationship had never been solid, and they eventually went separate ways. Alone in the giant megapolis with a handicapped child, Raia worked nights in order to be with Yana during
the day. Not withstanding her university degree, she cleaned rooms
at a school and supervised a girls' dormitory. She laboured endlessly
to teach her daughter to speak correctly. Ten years later, applying for
a job at a magazine, she met Volodya. They immediately fell in love
and married the following year in a civil ceremony.

We visit the Tver Regional Museum, with exhibits depicting the
natural and cultural history of the region. Raia is depressed that so
rich a heritage was completely destroyed by communism. The last
display, they warn me, is Soviet propaganda. We prepare to move
through it quickly, but suddenly, we stop short in astonishment. The
exhibit they remember from previous visits has been replaced by a
depiction of the Stalinist repression. It is the first time they have ever
seen this theme addressed in an exhibition, and the impact is almost
unbearable. It reminds me of exhibitions about the Nazi concentration camps—you can hardly stand it, but you force yourself to keep
looking and not to run away. We see photographs from the mock
trials and of deported prisoners, documents with their sentences,
death certificates. We see a replica of the steel prison door and of the
interrogator's table. We see a poster depicting Stalin as the "Father
of Orphans"—those same orphans whose parents he sent to die in
the camps.

Walking home, we are silent. I feel as if I have fallen down an
empty elevator shaft. Nothing in Russia is neutral, lukewarm, or su-
perficial. At every turn, you are plummeted to a new and unexpected
depth of suffering. But equally unexpected, equally extraordinary, is
the discovery, at the heart of the suffering, of the spiritual transcendence that is the particular quality of Russian culture and that has
enabled them to survive.

I hear it in Raia, who tries, haltingly, to articulate what is in her
heart. "Our sorrow is our richness. The photos of the prisoners—
they are like icons. Christ's Passion was not pretty either, but the
cross shone with light."

They ask me what I think. What do *I* think? What right do I have to think anything? And yet, because of Catherine and because of what she has given to us, because God is our life and because our vocation has come to us through Russia, I am not a stranger here. What I have been given is not just for myself, and with whom are we called to share this heritage if not with Catherine's own people?

Volodya translates for me: "What Raia has just said shows how this kind of suffering can be redeemed. What has happened through the centuries, what has happened under communism, what is happening now, all has meaning if we can lift it up to God in love and forgiveness. This is the meaning of the Resurrection, the victory over death."

What an awesome gift to be able to share these moments with them. No, among these people I do not feel like a stranger.

Monday, August 10 – Moscow

We got home late last night, and the phone was ringing. I don't know what time Raia and Volodya got to bed. I woke up during the night with severe nausea and diarrhoea. Raia says they always feel a little sick coming back from Lilia Stepanovna's, because her food is so rich. In my case, it's also fatigue.

I sleep most of the day, waking in the afternoon to take a phone call from Alvina Voropaeva in Magadan, in the far northeast of Russia. She says she has been trying to reach me for days. Alvina was the Russian interpreter for the Rotary Club group who visited Magadan in 1989. She is currently translating *Poustinia* into Russian; I met her when she visited Combermere last year.

Right now she is in a state of panic. At her invitation, Jean Fox and a senior staff worker, Marie Javora, will be coming to Magadan from Combermere in less than two weeks. They were to be Alvina's house guests, but now she has sold her apartment and doesn't yet have a new one. I can appreciate her predicament.

"Are you giving TV interviews?" she asks me. "Are you giving talks on Madonna House?"

I laugh. "No, I've just come to be with friends. To share their lives, to try to understand."

As a matter of fact, tonight Raia has arranged for some of the girls from the theatre group to come meet me and hear about Madonna

House. They were invited for five o'clock, began arriving at six, and we started talking at seven. Between the never-ending phone calls, Raia whipped together supper for ten: rice with cabbage and onions and a cake made from scratch. She pours in the ingredients without measuring, just as we learned to do in the Madonna House kitchen.

On top of the grand piano in Raia and Volodya's room, we spread out my Madonna House photos, the books by Catherine that they brought back from Paris last year, and the new MH literature in Russian. The girls are shy, so it is Volodya who feeds me with questions about Catherine's life, Madonna House life, and my own spiritual journey.

"Aren't you bored?" I keep asking.

"No, no!" comes the answer.

Seventeen-year-old Ira, who speaks English, tells me they only know Orthodox nuns with their veils and long sleeves and high collars. To them, the lay apostolate is a completely new form of Christian life. "You'll see," Volodya had promised, "she's like you. She laughs a lot. She's even pretty!"

Before we go in to supper, I spread out Catherine's shawl on the piano. We light a candle and each of the girls prays spontaneously. Although I can't understand the words, the sincerity is unmistakable.

At supper, I ask them to tell me about themselves and how they met God. They don't really open up until Volodya, tired from translating, asks Ira to take over. One of the most taciturn of the group decides to tell her story, after which they all begin to talk. I am amazed at the working of the Holy Spirit in their lives. For each, an encounter with Fr. Men had been a turning point.

Tuesday, August 11, 1992

This afternoon, I accompany Volodya to the Little Sisters of Jesus to visit Elena Vladimirovna, a Jewish-born woman who baptized herself on the eve of Easter when she was eight years old! At that time, she had had a powerful experience of God's presence. In the late 1930s, she and her husband were sentenced to the gulag for their faith. He perished in the camp. She was released during World War II and secretly became an Orthodox nun. In her old age, she joined the Little Sisters. She is now almost ninety and blind. We speak in French, which she, like most educated people of her time, had learned in childhood. I feel as if I am in the presence of a *staritsa,* a spiritual mother. She asks my age and where I have come from, but I am much more interested in learning about her.

"Please," I say, "tell me about your life."

"Such a long life! I am eighty-eight years old. How can I tell you?"

"Then tell me about God. Who is he for you?"

"What a question!" Then, "He is someone very far away and very near. All my life I have loved God. I am only now...sometimes...beginning to understand that he loves me."

Volodya, whom she adores, has brought his electric keyboard and plays for her the musical lament he wrote after Fr. Alexander's death. She too worked with Fr. Men for many years, and tears trickle down her cheeks as she listens to the poignant melody.

We have tea with the Little Sisters. They know the book *Poustinia,* and Sr. Claire, the superior, tells me that her father was baptized at our church in Paris. When we say good-bye, I ask Elena Vladimirovna to pray for me.

"Pray?" she says. "Sometimes I think I am a sceptic. Well, I will try."

Raia has a rehearsal tonight, so Volodya and I, leaving the Little Sisters', take the metro back downtown and then stroll through the older part of the city. The walls and towers of the Kremlin and the gilded cupolas of its churches are eerily beautiful in the dusk. Volodya talks freely, simply, about the effects of the political changes on his generation.

"The fall of communism is our victory and our tragedy. We have lost our enemy. But he was part of us, and without him, we don't know how to live. I thought I hated the Soviet Union, and now I realize it was part of me. Our generation is the most lost, for our best years are already behind us. We were unable to realize our goals, so we abandoned ourselves to our dreams. Everything is possible now—but we still only dream."

Moscow used to be the cultural centre of Russia, he says. Now it is a commercial centre to which everyone comes because there is money to be made.

He speaks of his alienation from his father and of the transparency of the communist lies. He talks of his student years when he and his sister travelled across Russia with their guitars, singing of God and of faith. Because remarks he had made in support of Baltic independence had been reported to the authorities, he was refused admittance to the Institute of Foreign Languages where he had wanted to study English. An earlier wrist injury had precluded the possibility of becoming a professional violinist. He ended up studying journalism and sociology.

It was of those early years of travels, dreams, and hopes that he had sung that night at his mother's, and which had resulted in such melancholy. "That world is gone," he tells me now. "We don't know who we are any more. Before, we suffered for our faith. I lost my job at the editorial board of the newspaper where I worked when they saw my baptismal cross and asked if I was a believer. Today, everyone from former communists to gangsters is a Christian.

"I used to understand this country. I knew how it operated, and I knew how to find my own life in it. Now I no longer understand anything. Each of our friends carries within himself terrible conflicts and contradictions. We have a love-hate relationship with Russia."

Wednesday, August 12 – Novaya Deryevnya

The weather and our hearts are heavy today as we travel by train and then by bus to Novaya Deryevnya, the village outside Moscow where Fr. Alexander Men's parish, and now his grave, are located. Raia buys flowers to place on his tomb. I have brought Catherine's shawl, but it seems too stagey to take it out of my bag.

The Divine Liturgy is being sung in the little wooden church, but we only stay for part of the service. The celebrant, Raia and Volodya tell me, is a priest who had been hostile to Fr. Alexander. For the Erokhins and their friends, the present reality of Novaya Deryevnya contrasts cruelly with their memories. The pastor, who was a disciple of Fr. Alexander, is on holiday and has taken with him the key to the memorial room so that the other priest won't dismantle it. During Fr. Men's lifetime, a second priest was always appointed to watch and report on his activities. Even after his death, the spiritual warfare continues.

When we go back outside, Volodya helps a group of young people who are building a baptistery, while Raia rests on a bench. I return to the flower-strewn grave to pray.

Catherine seems very close. I pray to her and to Fr. Men for Raia and Volodya, for all the people I am meeting, and for Russia. Into my heart comes the thought, *I know why I came to Russia. I came so that you could return, Catherine. It is time for you to come back to Russia. They need you here so desperately.*

We return on foot to the train station in the neighbouring town, following a path that leads past small farms. Volodya points out houses they used to visit with Fr. Alexander. He says Fr. Men showed him the face of God, but he doesn't have the strength to find God by himself.

"But God is in your heart!" I exclaim with unusual vehemence. I don't know why it matters so much to me. "Volodya, listen, you must believe! God is in your heart. He hasn't abandoned you. He will give you everything you need. He promised!"

"I've understood something today," Raia intervenes. "We have to come here more often. It's difficult for us, but this is a place of spiritual combat, and we have to fight for what Fr. Alexander started."

On the way home, I buy a rose for Raia. She says it is a dream-come-true. I could have bought a whole bouquet, but, out of respect for them, I don't want to be too profligate with money. It's absurd, but I've even been tormented about what to do with the suitcase of little items I collected for them from our house in Paris: toilet paper, soap, brightly-coloured pillow cases someone had given us just before I left, coloured aluminum foil I'd found on the street. There are also toothbrushes and toothpaste, little packs of Kleenex, bottles of aspirin and pain medicine, band-aids, and a few pieces of clothing.

Will these gifts offend them? Raia said to me a few days ago, "We don't have much, but we are happy," and only this morning, Volodya observed, "You came to us with just your smile and your heart."

Returning from Novaya Derevnya, I find a moment to call Raia into my room. I show her the gifts and try to explain the pain in my heart. As always, she understands.

"Miriam, you were afraid? You didn't have to be. You've seen how we live. These things are wealth to us. We are almost out of soap and I was wondering what to do. Now God has provided. We will keep what we need and share the rest with others."

She loves the pillowcases and coloured aluminum foil. The dish sponges are a treasure—she is finally letting me help with the washing up, but it is done in cold water, without soap, and using little scraps of greasy sponge. I've already given them maple syrup and honey from Combermere, coffee, two pretty tins of tea, a box of granola bars, and pâté. The last two items they are keeping for the bus trip.

This evening we have decided to unplug the telephone so that the three of us can be together in peace. I'd offered to take them to a restaurant, just to get away from the house, but Raia says Moscow is not like France—restaurants here are both expensive and unpleasant.

"Why don't we have a party ourselves?" she suggests. "We'll get a chicken, and we can have the chocolate and bottle of wine you brought."

But when we go to buy a chicken, there is not a fowl to be found in our end of Moscow.

"It doesn't matter," says Raia. "We can have rice."

I am learning something every day. My Parisian culinary education notwithstanding, what *does* it matter if we have chicken or rice? It's not the food that is important, but the time together, the sharing, the fraternity.

They burst out laughing when I ask which kind of wine they prefer, red or white?

"*Any* wine!' they exclaim.

"Do you realize," says Volodya, "we never relax like this. At least, not since things have become so expensive. Maybe that's why activity and rushing and primitive living become such a way of life."

Raia prefaces the evening by saying, "It has been a sad, heavy day. I want us to be cheerful!" Well, if what transpired could be described as cheerful, it must have been a distinctly Russian interpretation of the word. For me, it was the most intense of several very intense evenings we have spent together. Intensity must be part of the Russian character; they seem to live all the time with every fibre of their being!

Raia wants to know if I find it strange that they and their friends manage to live with humour when their lives are so hard. Do I see how difficult it is for them?

"Today, when I was shopping," she says, "a man was selling tomatoes. Many of them were rotten, but he said to me, 'Why do you have to pick them over? They're all good.' I threw them back and went and bought from someone else. This is an attitude we meet every day. People here have been slaves for seventy years. They've lost respect for themselves and for others."

At the laundry where they bring their bed linens and kitchen towels—their personal laundry they scrub by hand—the new linens they'd received as gifts in France had been stolen. Their number was re-sewn on worn, used items, and there was nothing they could do about it. Under the Soviet regime, this would have been a criminal act subject to severe punishment. Today they feel powerless before an increasingly lawless society.

Their own little group is different: Raia and Volodya, Olya Erokhina, Sonia, whom I'd met at Olya's and who had come this afternoon to pray in memory of Fr. Alexander, Elena Vladimirovna, and a wrinkled old woman we'd met at Novaya Deryevnya who had been sent to the camps for her refusal to condemn a fellow university student unjustly.

"We are the crazy ones," says Raia.

Do I think they can survive in their craziness? they ask.

I think they are like Blessed Basil, the Fool for Christ. Whether we come from the East or the West, we are all remnants in the biblical sense of the word. All of us are fools for God, fighting the brutality and perversions of our societies. I try to tell them about the terrible spiritual sickness of the West, but even though they have spent time in Europe, this is hard for them to grasp.

I love them both so much. They are crucified on the cross of their country. Tonight, once more, my heart is too full for words.

A cheerful evening?

Thursday, August 13, 1992

At the Tretyakov Gallery this afternoon, I realize that I am in a room with some of the greatest icons in the world, among them *Our Lady of Vladimir*, also known as Our Lady of Tenderness, and

Rublev's *Trinity*, in which the three Persons are represented as the angels to whom Abraham gave hospitality. The many reproductions I've seen of this icon do not begin to convey the beauty and harmony of the original or the incredible peace emanating from the faces. I am overwhelmed by the light streaming forth from the eyes of Rublev's *Saviour*. I don't know anything about icons except what they are now teaching me. Their presence transforms the museum into a church.

When Raia and I arrive home, Volodya and his sister Olya are using their English with Bro. Guillaume, a Dutchman from Taizé who has been living in Bangladesh for fifteen years. At the Danilov Monastery, where he has been staying, he has met with considerable unpleasantness because he is a Protestant. Tonight he leaves by train for St. Petersburg. Olya and Volodya have friends there and begin phoning to arrange a place for him to stay.

Raia leaves for a rehearsal. I watch Volodya gather food for Bro. Guillaume to take with him on the train. I know there isn't much in the refrigerator. Into a plastic bag Volodya places hard-boiled eggs, the tin of pâté I brought from Paris (and which they had been saving for our bus trip), apples, and a bottle of tea. Then Volodya drops into the bag a big chunk of the Belgian chocolate we'd savoured last night. They never get chocolate, and this brother is returning from Europe, where he has undoubtedly been feasted and feted to the hilt! Here they have so little, but they unhesitatingly give everything they have.

After seeing Bro. Guillaume off on the train, Volodya and I continue on another evening stroll. He shows me the Russian Parliament building, where he and thousands of volunteers outfaced the tanks during last summer's attempted putsch. Raia had been in Israel, and had the putsch succeeded, they might have found themselves permanently separated.

We walk to the Arbat, an old Moscow residential section. The street by that name has now become a tourist centre, but the surrounding neighbourhood retains its original character. The streets are empty. After work and grocery shopping, most people just go home, too tired for much else. Everything seems rundown, overgrown. Streets and more streets. Volodya shows me a beautiful circular courtyard he discovered by accident one day, when he was working in this area. We don't converse very much this evening.

Friday, August 14

I emerge from my room this morning to find Volodya trying to repair a dripping faucet. In the end, he has to call a friend to help him. I've washed my hair, and Volodya thinks I resemble Lily Brik, the mistress of Vladimir Mayakovsky, their famous poet of the 1920s. He and Raia talk about art and poetry and show me books of graphic art from the twenties. A new world of culture is opening for me.

Raia and I visit the eighteenth-century Sheremetyevo Palace, on the edge of the city, where a friend has arranged for us a private tour. I understand the gist of it, if not the details. Vespers in the adjacent church are beautiful, but Raia is visibly uncomfortable in the ultra-Orthodox atmosphere.

I am seriously concerned about Raia. She is so exhausted that I think she is on the edge of a breakdown. I mention it to Volodya this evening when we go walking.

I treasure these evening promenades. I've seen an amazing amount of Moscow this way, and it serves as an opportunity to ask questions, to exchange, and to learn—in English. Tonight he asks me if I would like to live in the U.S. again.

I am embarrassed. "I'm different from most Americans," I tell him. "In the 1960s, many of my generation disagreed with the policies of our government and felt alienated from our own country. I've never particularly identified with the U.S. and its culture. Then too, Madonna House is my real home, and ours is a culture centered on the Gospel. Does this make any sense to a Russian?"

He compares it to his own sense of alienation. "You need to be strong to live in Russia," he says. "I no longer understand anything about this country. I have to find myself again."

Saturday, August 15, 1992

While we were out last night, Teresa phoned from Paris. This morning we finally connect. She wants to wish me a happy feast of the Assumption and suggests that she meet me in Taizé on August twenty-third.

"You see the difference between Russia and the rest of the world?"
Volodya says to his wife. "Teresa says she'll be in Taizé on Sunday in
a car, and she will. It is simple. We say we will be there in a bus, but
who knows if it will happen? Will the bus come? Will it break down?
Will there be gas? Will the drivers run out on us?" And turning to
me: "Miriam, *this* is life in Russia!"

Today is the feast of the Assumption. Since the Orthodox liturgical
calendar is thirteen days behind that used by the Catholic Church*,
and since I have decided to live totally in Raia and Volodya's world,
I was not expecting to attend Mass. Their suggestion that we go to
the Divine Liturgy came, therefore, as a little gift from God.

Theoretically, the downtown Church of Sts. Cosmas and Damian
has been returned to the Moscow Patriarchate, but since the printing company that occupies the premises still hasn't moved out, the
liturgy is celebrated in a small, second-floor room. Adjacent rooms
are used for offices, storage, and classrooms. In one of them Volodya
teaches music to the children on Sunday mornings. To accommodate
all the people at the Easter Vigil, he tells me, they broke the lock on
the printing workshop and celebrated the liturgy amidst the typeset-
ting machines. Jesus broke out of the tomb, and they broke in!

We have been fasting since midnight. Volodya says that in this
parish, permeated with Fr. Alexander's ecumenical spirit, I can receive Holy Communion even though I am a Catholic, but that I
must first talk to the priest. I try to get him to be more specific. Is it
confession, or am I just asking permission? In retrospect, I should
have known it was the sacrament when the priest placed his stole
over my shoulder. "Yes," he says, "I can receive communion, but…"
I can hardly hear what he is murmuring, much less understand the
Russian words. Thinking the word for "sins," *grekhi,* means "Greek,"
I tell him how much I love the Byzantine liturgy! He must have ab-
solved me from pure desperation. Totally mortified, I forget to ven-
erate the cross and the Book of the Gospels, and have to be pushed
back in the right direction. There are other awkward moments. It is
one thing to be Catholic, but do I have to be so *stupid?*

---

* The Julian calendar was universally used in Russia until 1917, when the Gregor-
ian calendar was adopted for civil use. The Orthodox Church continues to use the
older form.

Such faux pas notwithstanding, I am moved at the core of my being. It is an incredible privilege to be able to share the Body and Blood of Christ with this living, resurrected Church. Compared to the splendour in the great cathedrals, the liturgy celebrated in this little room, with a choir of five, is simple and humble, but it is still the Divine Liturgy in all its depth and transcendence. I am so grateful to God and Catherine and Archbishop Raya for the immense gift of being able to pray this liturgy as my own, even without knowing Church Slavonic.

In the evening, I accompany Raia and Volodya to a rehearsal of the *Mystery of the Passion*, which they will be presenting in Germany. This is the first run-through with costumes and music, which was written by Volodya and performed by him and Olya. In addition to singing, they accompany the narrative on the violin, flute, percussion, and clarinet. The text is read by a narrator, and the overall effect is hauntingly beautiful.

I watch Raia work. She is an exacting director, and I am amazed at the energy pouring forth from her. Later she tells me that the young people lack discipline and commitment. The work is draining, and she wonders if the fruits are worth the fatigue and frustration. What strikes me is that she and Volodya are forming these young people by teaching them discipline, creative expression, solidarity, and faith. Once a month, they gather just to pray.

Sunday, August 16, 1992

We didn't go to church today, since Raia and Volodya seem to take it for granted that yesterday's attendance was sufficient. Even had we gone, they said, we would not have received communion two days in a row. However, we'd brought home pieces of blessed bread that we consume before breakfast, after saying grace.

Volodya takes me to see the Kremlin. At the entrance, a guard informs us that Russians are not allowed to go in this way. "I'm accompanying an American," Volodya snaps, and we are waved through.

Most interesting for me are Volodya's impressions. The Kremlin, he tells me, reflects the history of Russia—the splendour of the tsarist court, neglect after Peter the Great moved the capital to St. Petersburg, and then the oppressiveness of the communist regime. He always used to avoid coming to the Kremlin, but now the overhanging evil he always used to sense here has completely lifted. He is dumbfounded at the difference in the cathedrals, all of which are undergoing restoration. It is like seeing a resurrection.

I convince Raia and Volodya that I will be happy to stay home alone tonight while they are at the rehearsal. It is a chance to boil water for Tuesday's bus trip and to iron some of the clothes drying in the bathroom. Not used to heating the iron on the stove, I burn the collar on one of Volodya's shirts. Later, as I reorganize and pack my own belongings, I discover two miniature bottles of Canadian rye that Teresa hid in my suitcase. I set them on the kitchen table with little vodka glasses from the cupboard. Raia, returning after midnight, almost bursts into tears when she sees it.

"You *will* burst into tears when you see what I did to the shirt," I warn her, but she isn't concerned. To relax together after an evening of exhausting work is an unexpected treat for them. Thank you, Teresa!

Monday, August 17, 1992

Our departure is set for 7 A.M. tomorrow morning, and this is a day of preparation. I iron until Raia is ready to go buy food for the three- or four-day journey. At the closest government food store, it is a shock to find empty display cases and shelves. We try another store, about a ten-minute walk from the first. Here they have food, but the lines are long, and Raia, on principle, refuses to spend her time waiting. She buys meat, a real luxury, and we stop at kiosks on the way home for overpriced potatoes, tomatoes, and apples.

By evening, we are completing the last preparations. Sonia has come to spend the night. She worked with Fr. Men as a choir director, Sunday school teacher, photographer, and translator. Now fifty-eight and in poor health, she is still brimming with talent and interested in everything. She speaks slowly and clearly. I am comfortable with her.

As the two of us eat supper by ourselves, I hear Raia's raised voice coming from the bedroom. She is talking to someone on the phone, and her tone is unusually harsh and angry. A few minutes later, she and Volodya come into the kitchen to tell us the departure has been postponed until Tuesday evening. No explanation was given to them. They don't know how to contact the drivers; they don't even know who they are or from where the bus has been rented. All along, they have been uneasy about these arrangements, fearing last minute complications and even that the drivers might abscond with the money that was advanced to them.

I've never seen Volodya so furious. He keeps repeating to me angrily, "*This* is Russia!" Raia has a sense of foreboding and is ready to cancel the whole trip. There is more, but I can't follow, and this is no time to ask unnecessary questions. They return to their room to phone the other thirty-six travellers and inform them of the change in schedule. Soon Raia comes to tell us wearily, "It's getting worse and worse. Now Volodya and Olya are quarrelling."

Division is a sure indication that the evil one is mixed up in this, but I'm reluctant to say anything, aware that this is only one episode in their continuing struggle to carry out plans and fulfill dreams. How I wish I could speak more fluently! Since I can't, I just pray for spiritual protection. Going into the bedroom to fetch my rosary, I am moved to find Sonia on her knees before the icon. She says to me, "You know, I'm terribly sorry for Volodya and Raia—but frankly, I'm glad we can all get a good night's sleep!"

Finally, we all go to bed. Volodya has to be up by 6 A.M. to give the rest of the money to the bus drivers.

Tuesday, August 18

Since we now have a free day, Raia and Volodya decide I should see the Donskoy Monastery. I assent, since this will at least get Raia out of the house. While waiting for her to get ready, I have a lovely visit with Sonia, who, in the middle of last night's crisis, had begun asking about poustinia. What a gift this would be in Moscow, where people are so perennially tired and over-stressed.

At the monastery, any illusion that I am finally beginning to follow conversations is dispelled by our encounter with a monk who is angry that I am wearing a cross while dressed in an open-necked, short-sleeved shirt. Not understanding the words, and thinking he is interested in my cross, I smile broadly and begin explaining that "Pax-Caritas" means *mir i lyubov*. I am shocked by Raia's curt tone as she answers him. The next thing I know, he is saying shortly, *"Zdrastvuitye!"*—"How do you do?" and Raia hurries me off. I wonder if she is just out of sorts. Not until we are on our way home does she explain that the priest wasn't welcoming me, but insulting me! She told him, "This is our guest from France; the least you can do is to greet her cordially!"

Raia herself is wearing wide-legged slacks, and our heads are uncovered. Had I realized my blouse was inappropriate, I would have dressed differently out of respect for the monastery and for the cross I wear.

Upsetting as it was, the incident is overshadowed by our amazing encounter with St. Nicholas. Sonia had drawn a map to help us locate the miraculous, perfume-exuding icon in one of the little chapels of the monastery cemetery. We can't find it, and after our experience with the monk, Raia isn't about to ask for help. We turn to leave—and suddenly, just before us is St. Nicholas! We can even smell the perfume!

In awe, we pray. I didn't know St. Nicholas was the Russian patron of travellers. We definitely need his intercession.

At 4 P.M., laden with luggage, sleeping bags, water bottles, food, books, theatrical costumes, props, and musical instruments, Raia, Volodya, Sonia, and I head for the metro. At the last station, on the outskirts of Moscow, we are to meet the rest of the group and—hopefully—the bus that will take us through Russia, Belarus, Lithuania, the district of Kaliningrad, Poland, Germany, and finally to Taizé in France.

"OUR AMERICAN!"

Departure

No one is surprised when the bus is late, but as time wears on, I too begin to wonder if it will come at all. While waiting, we gather in the parking lot to sing First Vespers of the Transfiguration, which the Orthodox Church celebrates on August nineteenth. I can't help thinking how astonishing it is that we can do this publicly. Just five years ago it would have been unimaginable.

"The old days are gone," one of the teenagers tells me contentedly. Sonia, who belongs to another generation, shakes her head. "It isn't that simple," she says enigmatically.

When it starts to rain, forty people make a beeline for shelter in the metro station, dragging their bags awkwardly behind them. Volodya and his sister Olya are trying to find out about the bus.

"Could this happen in France?" Volodya demands, not expecting an answer. "A bus that is three hours late?"

He says it might come tonight, tomorrow, or not at all, but it finally appears at 8:30 P.M. By the time all the baggage is stowed and we are off, another hour has passed. But we have made it out of Moscow!

About half of the forty passengers are members of the theatre group. Most are in their late teens or early twenties, many of them students. All have come into the church through Fr. Alexander Men. They are all talented.

Sonia, with whom I share a seat, is the unofficial spiritual leader of the trip. Having directed the choir for fifteen years under Fr. Men, she knows the liturgy inside and out. She has been to Lourdes and Lisieux, passionately loves the Little Flower, and would give anything to be able to make poustinias. In Moscow, she shares an apartment with her alcoholic son, who beats his wife when he has been drinking. She comes to the Erokhins to get away. In the course of the trip, we often pray together.

The remaining passengers are either parishioners at Sts. Cosmas and Damian in Moscow or from Fr. Men's former parish at Novaya Deryevnya. Raia and Volodya know some of them well, others not at all.

Though people have brought their own provisions for the trip, we eat our meals together after singing the "Our Father" and blessing the food. Raia is constantly passing food from where she and Volodya are sitting to where I sit with Sonia. They are always concerned that I have enough to eat.

In the beginning, there is plenty to eat. Raia even brought a roast, which we are careful to consume the first day, lest it spoil. There are hard-boiled eggs, tomatoes, cucumbers, and cheese, though we end up giving most of the latter to Sonia, who can eat only dairy products, when her own supply runs out. We have apples, a bag of Russian cookies, and a box of granola bars I brought from France. There is also a tin of French pâté and a large can of Spam. Everyone has brought boiled water. Only when we reach Germany will it be safe to drink the water from the taps.

The woods serve as a public toilet. Late at night, as we make our first bathroom stop, someone calls out, "Boys to the right, girls to the left!" I laugh to myself at hearing this familiar directive in the middle of Russia. As Raia and I push our way through the bushes in the dark to take our places among the rows of squatting women, the scene strikes me as comical. No one seems in the least self-conscious.

Day One

Today is the feast of the Transfiguration, and we pass around a container of blessed bread that someone brought along for this purpose. A group gathers in the aisle around Sonia and Volodya, and we sing the Office of the Transfiguration.

There is a lot of prayer on this trip, and we need a lot of prayer. We live by it. In the West, at crucial moments, we would probably pray charismatically; here I experience the power of liturgical prayer as a means of intercession, as if the whole Church is lifting our petitions to the heart of God. It is thrilling to see the naturalness and faith with which these young people sing the litanies, largely from memory, passing back and forth the few available books. Once again, my heart swells with gratitude for our Madonna House heritage, for the gift of familiarity with the Eastern liturgy.

From time to time, someone brings out the musical instruments, and before I know it, a whole ensemble has gathered in the aisle: two guitarists, a violinist, a flautist, a clarinetist, and recorder players. Russian classical music is followed by Taizé refrains, orchestrated for multiple instruments. This is indeed an artistic group!

Volodya, the unanimously-elected leader for the trip, has chosen a route that swings to the north across Lithuania to the province of Kaliningrad (formerly the German Königsberg), where we will cross the border into Poland. Although we have documents identifying us as a Christian cultural exchange group, he anticipates border complications and thinks it may be easier if we avoid the congestion at Brest, the main crossing point.

The Lithuanian border presents no problems. The guards are impressed by my much-stamped American passport, easily identifiable among the thirty-nine brand-new, red Russian documents. I am moved to find myself in Lithuania, where two of my grandparents were born.

By the time we approach the Kaliningrad border village of Bragratyonovsk, it is already dusk. Although there was some doubt about whether the crossing remained open at night, our drivers insisted on making a long detour for gas.

These drivers give us problems throughout the whole trip, balking at decisive points, refusing to work with us as a team. "It's always those who are paid the most who work the least," says Raia after a two-hour wait to change a flat tire that should have been checked the night before. Another problem, which becomes increasingly flagrant, is that two of the girls are becoming involved with the bus drivers, defiantly distancing themselves from the rest of us. There isn't much anyone can do about it, but it increases the stress.

About a kilometre from the Polish frontier, the bus comes to a halt behind a long line of vehicles, most of them buses and large trucks. Volodya and a couple of the men get off to investigate. Half an hour later, they return and gather us all outside the bus to explain the situation.

Forty vehicles are queued to cross a border that closes at night and on the weekend. The vehicles at the head of the line have already been waiting four days and nights. For us the implications are serious. We can wait our turn, but this could mean arriving in Taizé in the middle of the following week, leaving little time before the performance in Germany on September first. Food, water, and sanitary facilities all present difficulties. There is no place to sleep, except on the bus. Sonia's health is not good, and we have with us several children.

Since it is almost 11 P.M., the only thing we can do at this point is to organize ourselves for the night. The men arrange to take turns standing guard outside the bus to insure that nothing is stolen from the baggage compartments.

Volodya stops by my seat. "So now you can have another Russian adventure!"

His words sting. I don't want to live this as an adventure; I want to live it as one of them. But behind his remark lies an inescapable truth: personally, I have nothing to worry about. I am safe with them, I have no timetable, and one way or another I will be able to get back to Paris. Their predicament is entirely different; this is but the most recent example of the frustrations that have clogged their whole life. As much as I might wish to identify with them in this situation, the discrepancy is obvious. The pain of it is always in my heart as I watch and pray and wait with them during these forty tense hours at the Bragratyonovsk border,.

I try to lighten the atmosphere. "Maybe you should put on your play for the border guards," I joke.

Volodya stares at me blankly.

"American humour," I explain apologetically.

He looks at me for a moment. "Yes, Miriam, but American humour needs American conditions."

I find myself biting back tears. Just keep your mouth shut, I tell myself.

A few minutes later I feel Volodya's hand on my shoulder. He has brought a plate of food for me and a blanket to wrap around my legs, for I am too lightly dressed for the chilly night. He and Raia are exquisitely vigilant for my welfare, and this added kindness, in the midst of all their anxiety, brings fresh tears to my eyes.

Although I've noticed that Russians don't seem to touch each other much, I reach up and take his hand. "Please, don't be concerned for me. You have enough to worry about."

Day Two

It isn't at all certain that we will be able to cross into Poland here. The main crossing at Brest has been closed for several days— "renovations" is the official explanation—and this small border point is likely to be inundated by the diverted traffic. Local officials are becoming anxious, and it is possible that this crossing too might be closed.

Early the next morning Volodya, together with Sergei and Marie, who work with UNESCO in Moscow, go to talk to the officer at the crossing. Because of our documents, they hope we may be given priority. We quickly draw up a list of the children and sick people on the bus, convincing the teenagers to subtract several years from their real ages and encouraging everyone to maximize any health problems.

Two hours later, the delegation returns. They have been told to go to the city of Kaliningrad, forty kilometres away, to pay an ecological tax that will give them the right to apply for a pass to cross the frontier. It seems the city is short of money! Even then, there is no guarantee we will actually receive the pass.

In this kind of situation, everything is a matter of personal whim and relationships. Earlier, in Moscow, Raia had explained to me that Russians from time immemorial have never paid attention to laws. The Soviet system was intransigent and people learned to get around it any way they could, but through the use of force, it managed to impose order on everyday life. Now this order has broken down, and in the resulting chaos, people find themselves as helpless and as victimized as they were under the totalitarian grip.

Everyone contributes money for the ecological tax and for a taxi to take Volodya, Sergei, and Marie into Kaliningrad. There are no embraces as they leave, but a murmured *"S'Bogom,* go with God."

"Now we pray," Raia tells the group. It is noon, and we will not have news for at least three hours. We climb down from the bus and start walking up a side road. The queue of vehicles now stretches far down the road we came from. We find a sunny spot on the edge of a field and begin the Office to Our Lady. Since we are still in the octave of the Transfiguration, we sing the prayers of the feast. We sing an *akathist,* a long poetic prayer to the Mother of God. People from other buses stare at us curiously as they walk by. Some pause to watch, and some make the sign of the cross. An old village woman passing on her bicycle stops, and I see her lips moving in unison with us. She stays a long time.

We pray the rosary, a devotion unfamiliar to most Orthodox Christians, but which Fr. Men taught to his parishioners. We pray to Sts. Sergei of Radonezh and Seraphim of Sarov, to St. George the Dragon Slayer, to St. Nicholas the Wonderworker and Patron of Travelers, and also to St. Francis of Assisi. In the words of seventeen-year-old Ira, "The prayer today was heated!"

After we finish praying, we go into the village to look for food. Raia runs back to borrow money from one of the young people and returns just in time to buy the last loaf of bread. We need milk for Sonia, but there is nothing left in the dairy store except butter. In the little fly-infested market, we buy a kilo of cherries, measured into newspaper cones. Raia abandons her search for milk and lets herself be talked into buying apples instead.

By the time our Kaliningrad delegation returns, it is four o'clock. Marie bursts into the bus, crying, "We got it! We got it!" Raia runs out to meet Volodya. It is a first step, wrested by prayer and dogged determination. They had talked and talked with the mayor, who kept refusing to give them the pass. "Suddenly," they tell us, "we had the impression that a barrier had fallen. He took our money, signed the paper, and we got out before he could change his mind!"

All this while, I barely know what is going on. I don't catch most of what is being communicated, and only now and then do I ask one of the English-speaking people—anyone except Volodya—to fill me in on the essentials. I don't need to know all the details, and in a way, the absence of extraneous information helps me to pray. I hold on to my rosary. Early that morning, Volodya, glancing down as he passed my seat, had seen on my lap the paper on which he had typed for me in Church Slavonic the "Our Father" and "Hail Mary" the preceding summer in Paris.

He smiled briefly. "Good," he said. "You just keep praying."

The next step is to return to the head of the queue, present the pass to the officials, and ask for priority in crossing. But by now the officers have changed, and this morning's promise is worthless. There is one thin hope: for several days, a bus filled with children has been parked in a small space at the side of the crossing. If that bus gets permission to cross the border and pulls out, there is a possibility we can swing our vehicle into the empty space and be in a position to request clearance ourselves. Otherwise we will have to wait our turn. It could be days in coming, and the border might close at any time.

In the early evening, the young people gather again on the grass to pray and sing. We go around the circle, and each in turn expresses what the Transfiguration means to him. All I can think of is that Jesus appeared in glory to prepare his disciples for the darkness of the Passion. "We don't know what is going to happen here," I say, "but we know Jesus is Lord. We know God loves us. We know he is here, and that no matter what takes place, he is always with us."

Olya Erokhina and I stroll down to the frontier. There are two gates, about half a kilometre apart, between which pedestrians are allowed to walk. To the right is a big field of sunflowers; we pick them and eat the seeds right out of the centre.

On the road, the scene is becoming increasingly chaotic. By now there must be more than fifteen hundred people milling about. Near the crossing, townspeople have set up stands with luxury goods, cigarettes, and liquor. It is becoming dangerous for the women to walk alone, or even in groups, unless accompanied by men. Early this morning, as several of us were brushing our teeth in a clearing, a car pulled up beside us, and two drunken youths tried to convince us to get in with them. One of them was actually pulling on a girl's arm when a man from our group came up. The youths took off. In the evening, as a group of us were walking back from town, a man loomed up in the darkness and tried to put his arm around Ira. Volodya was just ahead of us, and when Sonia called out to him, the man faded back into the night.

As Olya and I make our way back to the crossing point, we suddenly realize that the children's bus is gone! The space is empty, and members of our group run to make sure no one else occupies it. Volodya browbeats our recalcitrant drivers into manoeuvring our vehicle through the crowd into the vacated spot. Another miracle! We still haven't made it through the border, but it is a sign that God is with us.

A villager offers us beds, clean water, and hot showers for a very moderate sum. Raia asks if I am interested, but I prefer to stay with the group. Sonia doesn't want to go either, but several others accept, including a lady with a handicapped son.

Another woman offers to sell us fresh milk at her farm, only a couple kilometres away. Raia, Volodya, Sonia, Ira, and I set off on foot. In one of those quicksilver Russian mood changes, to which I am becoming accustomed, we are suddenly almost light-hearted. Even Volodya, whose concentrated determination is pulling us through this crisis, seems relaxed.

In the farm courtyard, we fill two bottles with fresh, warm milk to take back and share a third bottle between us. How good it tastes! Another woman comes up and offers us the hot tea in her thermos, which she wants to refill with milk. It has been three days since any of us has drunk anything hot, and to me, it is paradise. Then we share a bottle of kefir, a fermented milk drink similar to yogurt, which I didn't like in Moscow but now find delicious.

We sit together on a bench in the softly-lit courtyard, sharing our simple pleasures, playing with the cats, happy in each other's company, happy in God's providence. Despite the uncertainties that still surround us, for these moments we are at peace.

Back at the bus, there is consternation when we realize some of the girls are not accounted for. Despite their fatigue, Volodya and the other men have no choice but to fetch their flashlights and go back down the road. Sonia leads the rest of us in a prayer to St. Anthony of Padua. He must have appreciated the ecumenical overture, for the flock is soon gathered in safely for the night.

In our new, more exposed location, toilet "facilities" are more problematic. A field now extends between us and the woods, and with such an influx of people, the ground is slippery with cow dung and human waste. Because there is no question of any of us going further away unaccompanied, we make the best of the situation.

Day Three

It is chilly again this morning. Volodya is scheduled to speak to the officer on duty when the border opens at 9 A.M., and at 8:30, the rest of us huddle together behind the bus and begin morning prayer. Just as attention begins to flag, Raia sees Volodya, Sergei, and Marie approach the captain.

"Quick, quick!" she cries. "Pray anything! Pray!"

We start the hymn, "It is Fitting and Right" and "Most Blessed Queen."

Marie comes running back and leaps into the bus.

"She's going for the pass! He's going to let us through!"

We can hardly believe it, but it is true! Quickly, we pile back into the bus. "Drivers! Drivers!" they call. With some difficulty, the bus is manoeuvred out of the narrow space; we pass the first barrier and pull to a stop before the second one. Here we realize that in our haste, we've left two passengers behind. Someone runs back to get them while we wait again for permission to continue on.

The permission is not forthcoming.

Grimly, Volodya takes his seat next to Raia.

"Would money help?" I ask quietly. "Dollars?"

Volodya shakes his head. "In Russia, it is always a question of relationships. Back there, the captain liked us. This major doesn't. When someone told him we were on a pilgrimage of prayer, he said, 'Good. Then stay here and pray.' So we will wait until someone else comes on duty."

Sure enough, half an hour later, a new officer opens the barrier, and we proceed to the last Russian customs post.

To keep things as simple as possible, Volodya had requested that we not buy any of the merchandise on sale at the frontier. We have no liquor, and we have prepared a list of all our currency. The Russian officer collecting our documents stares coldly from my passport photo to my face. We all breathe a sigh of relief when he turns to the next person. Then we get off the bus, unload our baggage, and wait some more. Another hour goes by. The officer returns and begins calling us, one by one, to retrieve our passports and re-board the bus. When he comes to mine, he frowns at the name and growls, "Where is your American?" There is a laugh as I push my way through, collect my passport, and quickly scramble aboard. On the bus, one of the girls hugs me.

"*Our* American!" she says warmly.

By one o'clock Friday afternoon, we are once more on the highway, crossing Poland. We still have two-and-a-half days of travel before us. It is after midnight when we arrive in Wrosclaw, where most of the group spend the night in a parish hall, and I am sent, with several others, to enjoy the hospitality of a Polish family. Even more welcome than the late night feast they spread out for us is a hot bath and the chance to sleep in a real bed.

Day Four

Our hosts wake us up at 8 A.M., feed us a breakfast as copious as last night's supper, and send us off with bags of food for the rest of the trip.

The German border proves to be tricky, and we only get through by forking over one hundred and fifty marks.

At a rest stop that afternoon, we accidentally leave behind one of our boys. Since the bus cannot turn around on the divided highway, we pull off to the side and wait, while Volodya and two youths jog back three kilometres to collect the laggard. At a second rest stop, we meet a group of young picnickers who recognize our Moscow license plates and greet us warmly in Russian. They are Russian Germans, Baptists, who have returned to their ethnic homeland and are evangelizing the Russian soldiers still stationed there. They ply us with Bibles, religious books, and chocolate bars for the children, who share them with the rest of us.

In the evening, we stop in a picturesque little town in upper Bavaria. A supper has been prepared for us in the parish hall, and the tables are laden with German sausages, cheeses, and pumpernickel bread, as well as beer, cold drinks, and snack foods. In contrast to the good manners demonstrated by the children earlier in the day, some of the young people sweep the leftovers into their bags.

We spread out our sleeping bags on the gymnasium floor of the Catholic school.

Day Five

Since we don't have time to stay for Sunday Mass at the Catholic church, we sing the Divine Liturgy in the bus, omitting only the Eucharistic prayers. Sonia, sitting next to me on my right, guides us through the rubrics, while Volodya, standing in the aisle to my left, chants the deacon's parts in his rich bass.

Things are now calmer, and I find an opportunity to chat with him about the trip.

"Was it anger that got you through?" I ask.

He shakes his head. "No, it might have seemed like anger, but I was absolutely calm. I was totally concentrated on not letting my attention relax. The only mistake I made was in believing the officer who promised to let us through."

"It was God's grace, a lot of prayer, and hard, unremitting work," I suggest.

"That's our whole life, Miriam. Now you understand."

As we approach the French border in the early evening, I remark facetiously that if France, "my" country, gives us trouble, I will turn in my residency card! We are all astounded when suddenly, we find ourselves on the other side without even having been stopped! Having become accustomed to the complexities of the East, I had totally forgotten about the border conventions of the European Community.

We are not in a different country—we are in a different world. In my heart are mixed emotions, and it will take me a long time to sort them out. These people have become part of me.

In the wee hours of Monday morning, we reach Taizé.

Arise, Go!

It was one of those rose-tinted evenings when the slanting, golden rays of the setting sun soften the stone facades of the tall grey houses along the Seine.

Paris at its most beautiful.

I stood on the bridge between Notre Dame and the Right Bank and felt as if I were already saying good-bye.

My years in France had seemed the culmination of my life in Madonna House. Our apostolic life was rich and deeply satisfying. I loved being surrounded by history and culture; I was writing and editing. During my holidays, I took advantage of the opportunity to travel in Europe, Israel, and to our house in Ghana.

I had been given everything I'd ever dreamed of. Why, then, was I so often filled with a sense of emptiness, of stagnation in my life with God? Why did I feel as if I had lost my spiritual bearings?

The time in Moscow had pulled me back into the centre of my being. It had taught me more about our vocation than I could ever have anticipated. Never had I felt so attuned to spiritual reality. Was this the reason I had found myself so unexpectedly at home in Russia, despite all the contradictions, tensions, and disorder I had encountered there?

This wasn't just one more experience to be filed away in my memory under "International Adventures." It had to be integrated into my life. When I asked God how to do this, he seemed to be saying, *"Open your heart and love more."*

To my spiritual director I wrote:

> What really happened to me in Moscow?
>
> Part of it was the discovery of a totally different kind of life than we know in the West, and of the way it forms people. What made it so deep and intense was that I *cared*. Caring is a type of commitment. My heart was opened at a depth I didn't even know was possible. The selfless giving of which I was so often the recipient fanned in me the desire to invest all my energy in learning to "love, love, love, never counting the cost."

Touching our apostolic roots in Russia has given me a desire to live our Madonna House life in a more radical way—a desire for poverty, for a greater detachment from material needs and from the need to control. I want to foster this new awareness and not settle back into a comfortable way of life.

Along with the journal of my trip to Russia, I sent a more personal letter to the three DGs:*

The Russians I met don't need to be "evangelized." They want to know they are not isolated and that we are willing to help them rebuild the faith that is theirs.

I see two real needs. First of all, the young people are searching for the connection between the spiritual and the everyday. The sanctity of everyday life—what we call "the life of Nazareth"—is what Catherine preserved from the heart of old Russia and what they are now being challenged to restore.

The second thing we have to offer is the poustinia. Given all the stress and fatigue and unremitting demands of daily life, I don't know how anyone can stay in touch with God without periods of silence and solitude.

From all I have written it is probably obvious that a major shift has taken place in my heart. If God wishes, I am ready to leave Paris.

Jean wrote back,

Yes, it is clear that God is preparing you. That you felt Catherine's presence so strongly is a sign that the Holy Spirit is singling you out for Russia at some point in the future. For the time being, however, you must not get distracted. Keep centered on the needs of the Paris house, and *pray, pray, pray.*

---

* DGs – Directors General of Madonna House, representing the laymen, laywomen, and priests.

I stood on the bridge, bathed in the radiant evening light, and wondered if I was out of my mind. Why would I ever want to exchange this loveliness for shabby, dilapidated Moscow?

Moscow? If Madonna House were to open a house in Russia, it wouldn't be in Moscow at all, but in Magadan, a city 7500 kilometres to the northeast on the chilly Sea of Okhovsk, built by Stalin to administer the slave labour camps of the region.

Because of its connection with the camps, Magadan had always been closed to foreigners. Even Russians needed special permission to go there. In 1989, when the restrictions were dropped, one of the first foreign groups to visit the city was the Rotary Club from Whitehorse, Yukon. A member of the group gave the book *Poustinia* to their interpreter, Alvina Voropayeva.

Alvina had been raised by a Baptist grandmother in a small city south of Vladivostok, but her childhood faith was all but eradicated by the atheistic Soviet educational system. Zealous by nature, she became a fervent communist until her first husband taught her to recognize the contradictions between the rhetoric she had internalized and the reality around her.

Her marriage ended in divorce, and when a second marriage also failed, Alvina returned with her younger son to Magadan, where she had spent part of her adolescence. Life was a struggle, but Alvina was a fighter. Eventually she found work as a translator for a geological institute. By the time the Rotary Club arrived, she was also interpreting for the foreign, mostly Protestant, missionaries who were beginning to pour into the city. Childhood memories began to stir, and when she read *Poustinia*, her life took a three hundred-and-sixty-degree turn.

Alvina wanted nothing more than to translate the book into Russian. At the invitation of Trudy Moessner, director of Madonna House in the Yukon, she visited Whitehorse and Combermere. In December 1991 she was baptised into the Catholic Church in the Madonna House chapel. The following summer Alvina arranged for Jean Fox and Marie Javora to visit the young Catholic parish in Magadan. I had spoken to her on the phone from Moscow just before their arrival.

Though the labour camps had been closed since the 1960s, to most Russians, the name "Magadan" remained synonymous with the Stalinist repression. They found it hard to conceive of ordinary people living in a place with such grim associations and where the climate and isolation further compounded the difficulties of everyday life. Both Jean and Marie had experienced a tangible spiritual oppression, even while they were overwhelmed by the warmth and the spiritual hunger of the people who received them. Magadan might be the "back door" to Russia, as someone put it, but it too was part of Catherine's homeland.

Marie wrote to me of the urgency she felt about opening a house there and added something to the effect that she'd be happy to be with me in Magadan, "should it ever come to that." It was a week before I could reread her letter without cringing.

Please, God, I begged, don't send me to Magadan. I'm not the Siberian type. It would be like going into exile from everything I love. I knew, though, that my likes and dislikes had no place in this scenario. If the Lord was indeed calling me to leave Paris, it was not for me to specify my preferences. God was extending to me an invitation. I could accept it or reject it, but I couldn't bargain.

Something was beckoning me, something that I wanted deeply and could not get for myself. As I stood overlooking the Seine, with the spires of Notre Dame glowing in the sunset, it came to me that the only way to have more was to have less. The only way to go further was to take the leap.

God said in my heart, *"Trust me."*

Sobornost

No sooner had I arrived in Combermere the next spring for the annual Directors' Meetings than I made a beeline for the little cabin where Jean lived.

"What's happening with Magadan?" I asked, after she had greeted me.

"If we go, I have you and Alma slated for the team, with Marie as director," she answered. "But first, we have to talk about it at the meetings. The whole family has to be united in this. We can only go if we have *sobornost.*"

Sobornost was a Russian concept Catherine had introduced into the spiritual vocabulary of Madonna House twenty years earlier. She described it as the unity of mind, heart, and soul to which the members of the community were called when important decisions had to be made that affected the whole family. The return of Madonna House to Catherine's homeland fell into this category.

By the time we finally got around to discussing "the Russian question," as Jean called it, the meetings were in their third and final week. That afternoon, each of us who had spent time in Russia was asked to share something of what he or she had experienced there.

Marie and Jean spoke movingly of their trip to Magadan the previous August. I spoke about Moscow. Two others talked about the pilgrimage they had made with an Orthodox group two years earlier, travelling down the Volga River and visiting monasteries and churches along its banks. Despite their disappointment at not being allowed to attend the installation of St. Seraphim's relics at Divyevo as originally promised, it had been nonetheless a journey into the spiritual heart of Russia.

These weren't travelogues. Each of us was speaking from a place deep in our heart, a place that had been touched and transformed by Russia. We were struggling to transmit an experience of God, a recognition of our apostolic roots, and the significance of all this for our spiritual lives and our vocations.

By the time the last speaker had finished, I could sense a change in the air. It felt to me as if each person at that meeting was being touched by the power of the experiences described. It was as if the Holy Spirit had come among us.

When the discussion turned to the possibility of opening a house in Magadan, the men, especially, were concerned about the economic and political instability in Russia. One of the priests expressed reservations about Madonna House, as a Roman Catholic community, establishing itself in a predominantly Orthodox country.

Usually reticent about speaking out in a group, I found myself rising to my feet.

"As we talk, what comes to me is a sense of confidence in our Madonna House vocation. It's not as if we were hard-core evangelists! We aren't going to Russia to 'convert' people, but to love and serve them in simple ways. Catherine has given us a love for Eastern Christian spirituality, and we live with the 'two lungs' of the Church. This is a reality, and it will bear fruit as long as we keep listening to the Spirit. We can't figure out everything beforehand. We have a lot to learn, and we are bound to make mistakes, but if we stay before God, at the heart of our vocation, he will show us how to move.

"In my heart," I continued, "is a desire to live our call to 'arise and go' in a radical way, without fear. Maybe we won't be able to do it. Maybe we'll even have to come home. But if we do go to Russia, we can't try to protect ourselves. We have to be ready to give everything."

"We will just be living our Madonna House life," said Jean quietly. "All that is needed is to help people reconnect with their Christian roots, to affirm and set free what is already there. Madonna House has been a repository of the faith that was ripped away from them in those terrible times."

Marie added, "In Soviet Russia, the ability to trust was radically broken. It is crucial that people be able to see others living a life of faith."

Fr. Pelton, the Director General of the priests, cleared his throat. "The clearest sign for me," he said, "is that we have an invitation from the Catholic bishop. What we need now is to work out a mandate with him.* I don't think this will be too difficult."

The room was still. The silence had a quality I had never experienced before. It was as if this time of deep, prayerful listening to God and to each other had not only swept away doubts and reservations, but also the barriers separating us from one another. The result was a unity in faith and trust that was clearly not of our own making.

Someone said softly, "I think we have *sobornost.*"

These will be my people

After the meetings, I returned to Paris. The opening of the new mission was scheduled for September, and in the meantime, I needed to tie up loose ends so that Teresa could take up the reins as director. Jean encouraged me to take my holidays with Raia and Volodya in Moscow again that summer and to learn from them as much as I could.

Not surprisingly, this second stay was quite different from the first. The previous year I had discovered a completely new world,

---

* Madonna House foundations are established at the invitation of the local bishop, with whom agreement is reached regarding the particular mission of the given house.

and now that world was soon to become my own. As I stood at a metro station one morning and watched the crowd stream past, the realization suddenly hit me, "These will be my people!"

Raia and Volodya's suggestion that we visit Divievo for the feast of St. Seraphim didn't work out, and when an alternative plan to go to the reopened monastery of Optina Pustin also fell through, it seemed to me that I was meant, once again, to simply share the daily life of my friends. It turned out to be a good preparation for Magadan.

The summer before, Raia had been reluctant for me to go out on my own. This time I went shopping, first with her, then independently. I learned to bring along plastic bags whenever I left the house, to compare prices, and to purchase on the spot anything that was reasonable since I might not come across it again. I found out that envelopes could be bought in the post office, and that everything from passport fees to utility bills were paid at a branch of the government bank. When Raia went to register my visa at OVIR, the government office that dealt with foreigners, I accompanied her to see how it was done.

When all the pre-1993 currency was recalled from circulation with only three days' notice, and with a ceiling on the amount that could be exchanged, I saw the impossible queues and mounting indignation as people tried to use up their soon-to-be-useless money. Essential goods could not be purchased, for some stores and vendors refused to accept the old bills, and change in the new currency was not yet available. When one vegetable seller started giving out change in tomatoes, people either stood gaping in disbelief or burst out laughing

The French pastor of the Catholic Church of St. Louis told me not to worry about a new law restricting the activities of non-Orthodox religious communities. "There are so many things to worry about in Russia," he said, "that if you start worrying now, you'll never stop!"

The shabbiness of Moscow struck me with renewed force. Paint was peeling and pavements were broken. At the same time, scaffolding and reconstruction could be seen everywhere one looked.

Volodya told me that in the past few years, two hundred and fifty Orthodox churches had been reopened in Moscow alone. As

we strolled through the city one Saturday afternoon, stopping in at
vespers services in one church after another, I felt as if the words of
the prophet Malachi were being fulfilled before my eyes: "From farthest east to farthest west, my Name is honoured" (Mal 1:11). While
the restoration was thrilling, I was appalled at the scale of deliberate
destruction.

One of the day-long pilgrimages organized by Volodya for
groups of parishioners took us to the town of Kolomna, two hours
from Moscow by electric train. Kolomna was a historical jewel, with
most of its buildings dating from the seventeenth century. On every
street were churches. Though only two were still in use, before each
of them Volodya led us in prayers to the patron saint. It was one
thing to stand before an iconostasis in an active church, another to
pray while surrounded by scaffolding and building materials, and
still another to invoke the patron of a church currently being used as
a warehouse. Most moving of all was to stand in the mud and pray
before the ruins of a church that had been converted to a factory and
now stood abandoned.

Two or three times a week, I accompanied Raia and Volodya to
liturgies at their parish of Sts. Cosmas and Damian. The year before,
services were still being held in a small, second-floor room. Now the
printing company had finally moved out, and the church, though
badly in need of renovation, was basically useable.

I was edified by the warmth and hospitality of this parish and
by the efforts of the two priests and a deacon to form Christian
conscience and community. They emphasized in their teaching the
incarnation of faith in daily life, repeating again and again, "To be
Orthodox is to be a witness."

When I introduced myself to Deacon Georgy and told him
about our soon-to-be-established Magadan foundation, he said simply, "Your presence there will be important for us."

The ecumenical spirit of Cosmas and Damian, which reflected
that of Fr. Men, was unusual among Orthodox parishes. At the
opposite end of the spectrum was a small church, dedicated to St.
Nicholas, where we took refuge from a rainstorm one afternoon
when we were walking in the city.

Vespers were being sung as we entered. As it was customary for
women to cover their heads in Orthodox churches, I had learned to

carry a scarf in my purse. I put it on now and stood quietly at the back, content to let the prayer wash over me.

A woman of about forty, dressed in black, was watching us. After a while she came over to me. "Are you a believer?" she wanted to know.

"Yes, of course," I replied.

"But you aren't Orthodox."

"No, I'm a Catholic."

She said something I didn't understand.

"Please, I would just like to pray," I said gently.

"Then you should pray correctly and cross yourself the Orthodox way!" she snapped and walked away.

I had been trying to feel out what was respectful and at the same time personally authentic in terms of my comportment in Orthodox churches. Covering my head seemed a simple courtesy, but I had continued to make the sign of the cross from left to right. Even though it identified me as a Catholic, why should I pretend to be anything else?

I told myself now that if I intended to live in this country, I'd better get used to these kinds of incidents. I tried to offer the pain in reparation for the sins of both Catholics and Orthodox. Wasn't it a matter of loving? And not just of loving the Christians at Cosmas and Damian, or the people with whom I could easily identify, but of loving those who rejected me?

Volodya had a different viewpoint, and it was categorical.

"Miriam, what happened today has nothing to do with authenticity. It has nothing to do with love. The way you cross yourself is part of a language. When you go into a village, you don't speak English if you wish to be understood. When you go into these conservative churches, it is as if you were in a different country. What you don't realize is that a war is going on between that country and yours, as well as with the 'country' where Raia and I live. We cannot make peace; the most we can do is to prevent an outbreak of hostilities. If you want to speak the Catholic language, you will need an interpreter to explain that you are just a foreign tourist. Otherwise, crossing yourself that way will be seen as a provocation.

"You cannot identify with those people. You are too different."

I went to bed that night filled with trepidation. How would we ever live in this country? It is too much, I thought. Russia is too much.

I asked Raia, "How do you deal with all the tension? It never lets up, does it?"

"You just have to keep living," she said.

Unexpected encouragement

On my return to Paris at the beginning of August, I continued preparing for my departure. One evening, Teresa and I invited Yves Hamant, the author of a highly acclaimed biography of Fr. Alexander Men, to have supper with us. A practicing Catholic who had been invited as a lay expert to the 1990 Synod of European Bishops, he had served as a cultural attaché with the French embassy in the Soviet Union and now taught at the University of Paris. From his unassuming demeanour, one would never have guessed the high esteem with which he was regarded for his expertise and knowledge of Russian affairs.

As we discussed the complexities of Orthodox-Catholic relationships in Moscow, I observed, "At least, we won't have the same conflicts in Magadan."

"You will find *exactly* the same conflicts there," he told us. He underlined the importance of us taking the initiative in contacting the Orthodox authorities, reassuring them that our purpose was not to proselytize, but to pray and serve.

As we said good-bye, Yves Hamant turned to me and said, "I'm always nervous when I hear about Catholic communities going to Russia. But having talked with you and Teresa this evening, I can truly say that not only am I reassured, but I'm genuinely happy that Madonna House will be in Magadan."

Madonna House in Magadan

It was close to midnight on September 23, 1993 as the half-empty Aeroflot jet from Anchorage rolled to a stop before the little airport in Magadan, Russia. Along with the other passengers, Marie, Alma, and I were herded onto a rickety bus and into the shabby terminal, where our nine suitcases were cleared by customs. Waiting to greet us with tears, flowers, and open arms was Alvina Voropaeva, accompanied by a lovely young woman named Lilia.

For three years, Alvina had been hoping, praying, and trying to persuade everyone, from the pastor of the Catholic parish in Magadan to the bishop in Siberia to the Directors General of Madonna House, that the spiritual family of Catherine Kolyschkine de Hueck Doherty was destined to return to their foundress's homeland through this unlikely door. Now Alvina could hardly believe it was happening. Nor could we!

Leaving the driver of the rented van to heave our suitcases into the back of the vehicle, we climbed in ourselves for the fifty-kilometre drive through the clear, cold night. Alvina chattered away in Russian, which only I could understand. Marie's Czech background and innate sensitivity compensated for her lack of formal study, but tonight she was far too tired to concentrate. And Alma, who had the most trouble with the language, was too busy looking out the window.

Entering the city, we turned onto Proletarskaya Street, one of the main thoroughfares. Unlike the tree-lined streets of Moscow, here were only a few scrubby little tamarisks. At this late hour, the street was deserted. The shabby buildings seemed utilitarian and bereft of beauty.

Our home for the next three weeks would be two rooms in a building in which the first three floors housed a bank and the fourth and fifth floors, a hotel. The hotel manager, a Catholic parishioner, had offered us the rooms without charge until we found an apartment.

A small but wiry night watchman helped carry our heavy bags up the four flights of stairs. Led by Alvina, we passed through a dingy lounge, where the woman on duty nodded to us, and down a dimly-lit hall to our rooms. These had been prepared with loving care by Alvina and other friends from the parish, who had brought dishes, cutlery, pots and pans, canned goods, and basic food stuffs. On a hot plate was a pot of soup, but we were too tired to eat.

Alvina and Lilia didn't stay long. We made up our beds, fitting the standard-size blankets into the Russian top sheets, and were soon asleep.

The next morning we awoke to sunny skies and a crisp temperature. Through the window, Alma and I had our first impression of this Stalinist city constructed of cement. In all directions rose five-storey buildings that had once been white. Nicely-dressed people hurried along the street. In the distance, on all sides, were the *sopkas,* which, someone had explained to us, were "higher than hills but lower than mountains." They were brown and grey in what was, for Magadan, already late autumn.

We were pleased that ours was a hotel for Russians rather than foreigners. The rooms were set up not only for sleeping, but also for eating and socializing. We designated one as a bedroom and the other for "living," and had just established some basic order when another of Alvina's friends, Rima, arrived with her nine-year-old daughter to show us around the city.

Our first stop, at the top of a long, steep street, was the Orthodox Church of the Holy Spirit. Sparkling white, with a blue tiled roof and a golden cupola, it seemed a sign of hope in this bleak-looking town. As we stood watching a baptism, an older woman in a black dress and kerchief came over to us, hugged Marie with obvious joy, then warmly embraced Alma and me. Responsible for everything from selling candles to singing the responses at the various services, she had met Marie the previous year and was delighted to see her back.

Outside the church we ran into Matushka* Fiokla, who also had befriended Marie and Jean the year before. Short and round, also dressed in black, Matushka had a high, little-girl voice and shining, childlike eyes. Her son, Nikola, struck me as a teenager trying hard to be an adult. The two of them were Old Believers, members of a

---

* *Matushka* – a dimutive for "mother," used by Orthodox nuns. It wasn't clear if Matushka Fiokla had actually taken vows, but in Russia, such fine points were often irrelevant.

group that had broken away from the Russian Orthodox Church in the seventeenth century.

Continuing along sidewalks with broken concrete, and manholes on which Rima advised us not to step, we peeked into stores along the way to see what was being sold. The windows gave no indication, and the identifying placards only read "Food" or "Merchandise." We took note of one establishment that sold different kinds of fish at what seemed to be reasonable prices.

Magadan is built on hills, and after a couple hours of climbing up and down, we were ready for lunch and a rest. Rima led us back to the hotel by way of Lenin Street, where the buildings, constructed by Japanese prisoners just after the war, were slightly more stylish. The tamarisk trees lining the street were already bereft of their needles.

Alvina had invited us to supper. Arriving at her two-room apartment, a five-minute walk straight up the hill from our hotel, we were surprised to find an elegantly set table and seven or eight other guests, all dressed up for the occasion. As Alvina hadn't given any indication that this was to be a welcoming party, we hadn't changed from the clothes we'd been wearing all day, but no one (except us) seemed disturbed by the discrepancy. All that seemed to matter was that we were here, and any shyness we might have felt was dispelled by the warmth of these women, all of whom were parishioners and friends of Alvina. Someone had brought a bottle of champagne, and there were repeated toasts to *Dom Madonny,* as Madonna House was called in Russian.

Buying an apartment

Since landlords charged higher rents to foreigners, whom they automatically considered wealthy, we had been advised to purchase an apartment. Alvina had been watching the newspapers, and after the meal, we went to look at an apartment she had seen advertised. Located in a neighbourhood built during the Stalinist years, the apartment had three spacious rooms with beautiful, built-in wooden cupboards, though the kitchen was small. We agreed that it was too elegant for us.

On our second day in Magadan, Lilia, the young woman who had met us at the airport with Alvina, took us to see another apartment, not far from our hotel. A burly man in his early thirties named

Nikolai came to the door and showed us around. This apartment also had three rooms, in addition to a toilet room, bathroom, and a medium-sized kitchen that was a definite improvement over the one we'd seen the previous evening. There was also a glassed-in balcony with clotheslines. Lilia explained to us that in the winter, balconies served as walk-in freezers and in the summer, as greenhouses. The apartment seemed to be in fairly good condition, with wallpaper that could easily be patched in the places where it was worn.

The best feature of all was still to come. We followed Nikolai outside, through a door beside the building entrance, down into the basement, and along a dark, winding hall to a sturdy, padlocked metal door. When he unlocked the door, we found ourselves in what is called a *podval*, an underground storage room. A trap door in the floor gave access to a little root cellar where potatoes and other vegetables could be kept.

It was a definite possibility. We headed back to consult with Alvina and then to look at the third address she had found in the newspaper. This one was located at the far end of town near Nagayevo Bay, where quite a few new buildings were under construction. We had trouble finding the apartment, and something in the atmosphere made us uneasy. As we stood on the sidewalk, trying to orient ourselves, a glass bottle came flying from an apartment window and crashed on the pavement near us. A minute later, a second bottle followed.

"I don't think this is the place for us," said Marie.

Back to Alvina's. She phoned Nikolai to tell him we would buy his apartment, and he agreed to meet us at her home the following evening to discuss the details. To say our heads were spinning would be an understatement. After all, this was only our second full day in Russia, and we were already on the verge of buying real estate. Marie, who would be signing the documents, could hardly write her name in Cyrillic!

We didn't have a clue about procedures. Could foreigners even buy property? Alvina phoned Lyuba, the parish administrative assistant, who assured us there was not a problem.

Sunday evening we met Nikolai at Alvina's, as planned. He agreed to wait until Thursday so that we could change our American dollars into roubles. When the three of us withdrew to the kitchen to confer in private and to pray for a moment before making the final decision, Nikolai thought we had gotten cold feet and were withdrawing from the agreement. Alvina interrupted our deliberations to tell us he was leaving, and Marie hurried out to stop him.

On Wednesday we changed sixteen thousand dollars into roubles, and the following day, Alvina took us to the notary's office, where Nikolai had been standing in line since 4:30 A.M. After waiting with him in a narrow, dimly-lit hall, we learned that since his wife was co-owner of the apartment, he could not sell it without her written authorization. She and the children were already settled in Ukraine; she could send the authorization by telegram, but it would require an extra day.

On Friday, we returned to the notary's armed with the telegram, but now the notary refused to accept Alvina's documents because her translator's diploma was made out in her maiden name and her internal passport in her married name. Alvina hurried home to phone a friend, also a translator, who arrived with her own diploma. Just before it was discovered that her documents had the same irregularity as Alvina's, Nikolai managed to switch us to a less exacting notary. We made a quick trip to another location to pay the sales tax, then returned to finalize the sale. Marie carefully signed her name in Russian, and we presented the second notary with the bottle of champagne that Nikolai had instructed us to purchase at a nearby kiosk.

Back at the apartment that now was ours, we gave a jubilant Nikolai his money, and he handed us the keys. Off he went, leaving the three of us and Alvina in Madonna House Magadan! We knelt in the room we had already designated as the chapel and said a prayer of thanksgiving.

For the next week we continued to live at the hotel while we scrubbed the apartment, whitewashed the ceilings, and shopped for some basic furniture. As the hotel was closing soon, we were able to buy from them, at a very low price, much of what we needed.

Magadan–the capital of Kolyma

The city of Magadan is located between two bays: Gertner, on the east, and Nagayevo, on the west. From the early 1930s until Stalin's death in 1953, Nagayevo Bay served as the gateway to the

Kolyma region for over three million prisoners sent there to work and to die. For the first few years after our arrival, everything we saw seemed permeated with these associations. Tree stumps on the hills were reminders of the women who felled birches and pines in winter temperatures as low as minus fifty Celsius. The Kolyma highway, stretching north from the centre of town for more than a thousand kilometres, was a silent testimonial to the convict labourers who had died at the rate of one every ten metres. This highway was literally built on bones. Our apartment building stood on the site of a former women's camp.

In the centre of the city, a giant statue of Vladimir Ilyich Lenin loomed over a vast square flanked by an uncompleted, sixteen-storey concrete structure. This was to have been the new Communist Party Headquarters. Seven years later the statue would be quietly moved to another location and the whole building dismantled down to the second storey, which became the foundation for an enormous Orthodox cathedral.

Magadan had been the regional administrative and educational centre for the many villages spawned by the gulag and surviving its demise.* Beginning in the 1960s, special benefits were offered to those who would brave the climate and isolation to help develop the Russian Far East. Thousands of geologists and other professionals responded. By 1989, the population had reached 152,000.

After the collapse of the Soviet Union, the central government could no longer afford to subsidize the region. By the time we arrived in 1993, hundreds of families were leaving for the "continent," as Magadaners called western Russia. We often saw big freight containers parked outside the apartment buildings, waiting to be filled with furniture and other possessions, including automobiles. The container would be shipped by sea to Vladivostok and then by train across Siberia. We would also see trucks coming from the Kolyma Highway, heavily laden with the belongings of those moving to the city from the dying towns and villages of the outlying areas.

---

* Political prisoners began to be freed after Stalin's death in 1953. After 1954 most of the Kolyma enterprises were converted to free labour, with the exception of penal colonies for criminals.

Settling in

Our own five-storey apartment building was sheltered from the din of traffic on busy Proletarskaya Street by two buildings identical to ours, separated from each other by dilapidated courtyards. From the kitchen window we could see a large, government-run childcare facility. Behind us stood Middle School #30 and the Municipal Choir School. More apartment buildings stretched on into the distance, flanked by hills and mountains.

Our building had four entrances, with each entrance giving access to fifteen apartments. This was a typical arrangement, although some buildings had four, rather than three apartments on each landing. There might be a three-room apartment such as ours, a two-room apartment on the other side of the stairwell, and one or two single-room apartments between them. Even the one-room apartments had a separate kitchen, toilet, and bath.

Despite Russia's enormous expanse, there had always been housing shortages in the cities. Each person was officially allotted fifteen square metres of living space, with a surcharge for extra space on the monthly "rent" collected for building services by the *Domaupravleniye,* the department that administered all state-owned buildings. Many families still inhabited communal apartments, in which an entire family lived in a single room and shared kitchen and toilet facilities with those occupying the other rooms. People were used to living with little privacy or personal space; it was a rare child who had his own bedroom. Often the parents would sleep on a pull-out sofa in the living room, storing their clothes and bedding in the drawers and closet of a tall three-piece cupboard set that stood along an inner wall of the room.

Considering that we almost daily came home laden with purchases, we were fortunate that our apartment was located on the second floor. The largest and sunniest room became the library-living room. Instead of the usual sofa and cupboard set, we put two tables together in the center of the room with chairs around them. Later, when we discovered a small furniture factory, we ordered standing book shelves, which came to line the walls as our Russian library grew.

The next room, which opened onto the balcony, was slightly smaller. There we fit our three beds and bed-stands, a wardrobe with shelves and a small hanging space for clothes, and a big wooden desk. Here the three of us slept and did office work. We delighted in such distinctively Russian items as the sets of drawers on wheels that fit beneath the desks, and the blankets that fit inside sheets. Any clothes we weren't using were stored in suitcases at the foot of our beds; under the beds were pull-out cardboard boxes designed by Alma. When we visited Russian homes, we were always impressed at the way people kept their personal belongings out of sight, and we tried to emulate their tidiness.

In the third room we set up the chapel. This, the spiritual heart of our house, took shape gradually over several years. We eventually replaced the blue-patterned wallpaper with one that was off-white and textured, and the Formica table with a simple wooden altar built to specification at the Magadan furniture factory. We found an Oriental rug for the floor and drapery material that went with its colours. For a long time, I found it hard to pray before the framed paper icons of Our Lord and Our Lady on the wall on either side of the crucifix. Although they were reproductions of the icons that had hung in St. Seraphim's cell, I disliked the Western European style characteristic of nineteenth century iconography. By the time one of our friends commissioned real icons for the chapel, however, I had learned to see beyond the aesthetics.

Our move from the hotel took place on October ninth. A Canadian we had met through Alvina helped us load our bulging suitcases and the furniture we had bought from the hotel into his big Ford pickup. The first snow of the season had started to fall. He made a second trip to collect the furniture we'd bought from a parishioner who was moving to Moscow.

Thrilled to be in our own home, we each went to bed that night with a sleeping bag, two blankets, and a pillow case stuffed with whatever was at hand. But just as we began to relax into sleep, we were jarred awake by loud music coming from below, so loud that the beds vibrated beneath us. No earplugs could deaden the noise, which continued until almost 4 A.M. This was to be part of our life, night after weary night, for the first year.

The previous year, when Alvina had unexpectedly found herself unable to host Marie and Jean in her apartment, Ella and Vasily Ostapenko, who were TV journalists, had opened to the two North

Americans their home and their hearts. The visit had changed the Ostapenko's lives, for they saw in Jean and Marie the incarnation of God's love. Marie and Jean, in turn, had been overwhelmed by Ella and Vasily's hospitality and by their spiritual hunger. The ensuing friendship, which came to include Alma and myself, was extraordinarily deep.

Russian furniture comes in pieces, and each time the furniture is moved, it is taken apart and reassembled. Ella and Vasily put together our beds, tables, and wardrobes. They and their good friends, Dima and Zhenia, spent entire weekends helping to make the apartment comfortable and attractive.

Elbruss, named for the highest peak in the Caucasus mountain range, was another of Alvina's numerous acquaintances. He was a geologist at the institute where Alvina had worked as a translator. He and his colleague Tatiana appeared at the door one day to offer their services for anything we might need done. Elbruss set about assembling the kitchen cabinets we had found at the furniture store, while Tatiana, a talented seamstress, made the drapes and tulle "inside curtains" for our apartment.

A freelance English teacher came up to us at the first parish Mass we attended and offered to help us in any way she could. Inna proved to be a treasury of background and practical information. She became our guardian angel, with a knack for showing up just when we needed her.

Our first crisis occurred not quite a week after we moved into the apartment. We had been scrubbing everything in sight, unaware that each time we emptied our buckets into the bathtub or kitchen sink, the water gushed from a broken pipe behind the wall directly into the newly remodelled kitchen of the neighbour below us. The neighbour was very kind about it, probably because we were *amerikantsy* and didn't know better. Inna phoned the maintenance section of the *Domaupravleniye,* and she too emphasized that we were Americans. Apparently, this was the only way to get a response, as the agency was concerned that foreigners did not receive a bad impression.

The following day, two not-quite-sober men rang the doorbell. They spoke so fast that at first, we didn't realize who they were, but Inna appeared just in time to identify them as the repairmen we were expecting. They fixed the pipe the next day with only minimal damage to our kitchen wall.

On November ninth, exactly one month after we had moved in, our parish priest, Fr. Austin Mohrbacher, celebrated the first Mass in our little chapel. He installed the Blessed Sacrament in the small wooden tabernacle, which had been so lovingly constructed for us by our Madonna House brothers and which we had brought with us from Combermere. Alvina happened to come by just in time to join us.

When we went to sleep that night, we could see from our beds, through the open door, the red glow of the electric tabernacle lamp. The Lord's presence in the Blessed Sacrament was a gift for which we were continually grateful, and we experienced its protection and power in our own lives and in the lives of those who came to us. Adoration of the Blessed Sacrament, together with the Eucharist, was our main source of spiritual strength.

Learning to live in Russia

From our first day in Magadan, when Rima and her daughter came to take us around the city, it was obvious that the Lord meant us to become intimately involved with his people. It was equally obvious that if our house was to truly have an open door, and if we were to truly embrace each person who came to us, no matter what the hour of the day or night, then God would have to enlarge our hearts. For each of us the process would involve a unique spiritual journey.

The starting point was in responding to the call of each moment. When people came to the door, we invited them in. If we were eating, we set another plate and pulled up another stool. Between meals, we poured countless cups of tea and brought out whatever sweets we happened to have. Our visitors never came empty-handed: they would bring a chocolate bar, baked goods, a bag of sugar, perhaps pillow cases or something else they thought we might need. Alvina had told them how we lived at Madonna House, but we learned it was a Russian custom to arrive with a gift, however small.

From our friends we learned how to live in Russia. We had to be taught everything: how and where to shop, how to seal our windows against the icy winter winds, how to freeze cowberries, called *brusnika*, on the balcony for winter vitamins, and where to pay our monthly bills. Lyuba, Fr. Austin's secretary and assistant, guided us through endless administrative procedures.

We continued to invest considerable time and energy in looking for supplies and furniture. For many items it was hunt-and-go-seek. The whole city was in a state of flux, and our friends didn't know where to find things either. Simply locating toilet paper could be an achievement.

People appreciated our desire to eat as they did. Inna came to help us salt cabbage for sauerkraut; others showed us how to make Russian dishes such as borscht, meat or fish cutlets, and *pelmeni*, a Siberian specialty something like meat dumplings. Ella brought us dried seaweed—"sea cabbage," as it was called in Russian—and showed us how to reconstitute and prepare it. She said it was very high in iron and an essential supplement to our diet.

Ludmilla, a pharmacist, would often drop by to see how we were doing. Though we enjoyed watching the courtyard from our kitchen window, it bothered her that we had no curtains, and others could also look in at us as well. One day she came and measured the windows, returned with a brightly-printed fabric, looked again at the windows, and left. When she arrived the next day, she had sewn us a pair of kitchen curtains!

Tanya Kononova and her nine-year-old son Kirill were frequent visitors. Kirill served as an altar boy at Mass. The previous year Tanya had arranged for him to help a friend distribute humanitarian aid through the parish, so he would "see how other people had to live." Peeking in while Mass was being celebrated, he thought he saw a ring of light surrounding Fr. Austin. Some months later, Kirill asked to be baptized in the Catholic Church. His mother and older brother soon followed. Tanya taught at one of the elementary schools and had won an award as the best teacher in the city. She often stopped in to help us with our Russian.

It wasn't long before Veronika and her daughter Nelly, a doctor, invited us to the two-room apartment where they and Nelly's two teenaged daughters lived. Nelly's husband had been murdered the previous summer. Veronika, a Lithuanian, had been brought to Magadan as a political prisoner in 1949. Throughout those terrible years, she had been sustained by her deep Catholic faith. "Of those days, there are no happy memories," she told us flatly. She had emerged from the camps with her health permanently damaged, but neither age nor infirmity nor blizzards nor icy sidewalks could keep Veronika from attending Sunday Mass.

Nina and Nadia were half-sisters. They stopped by often, as the music school they had co-founded was just behind our apartment building. Nadia was the director, while Nina coached vocalists. Her choir of upper-grade students sang at the Sunday liturgies.

After Mass one Sunday, Nina invited us to lunch at her apartment. I described the visit in our diary:

> They took us by bus to Nina's one-room apartment in an outlying neighbourhood. She has two sons, one of whom lives with his wife and children in St. Petersburg. The second, Toli, lives with her. He is eighteen and will soon be joining the army. In the meantime, he has tacked up posters of nude women all over the walls of their living room.
>
> Nadia is married to a ship mechanic, who spends months on end at sea. The boats are stuffy, and small enough to be tossed by the waves. Even when they are in harbour, many of the men live on the ship—their families are in other towns, and they lack the money to join them. They aren't receiving their salaries, but from time to time they are given a desultory amount, which they spend on drink. "And so, these strong, healthy young men are turning into alcoholics," said Nadia.
>
> When we got off the bus and headed for Nina's apartment, Nadia made a quick detour to pick up some chicken for lunch. With utter simplicity and a total lack of self-consciousness, she and Nina put the meal together while we looked on with avid interest, crowded into the tiny kitchen along with the dog and cat.
>
> Nina apologized that she had only forks and spoons and a combination of different-sized plates on which to serve the meal, which was accompanied by a bottle of Moldovan wine.

She is fifty-three and past the retirement age,* but works two jobs because, with inflation, her pension is not sufficient. People keep telling us that everyone is becoming poor in Russia.

Though clearly exhausted, Nina begged us to stay as long as we could. "There's something pure coming from you," she said. "It is so restful to have you here. It's so easy to relate to you!"

Each person we meet, each person we come to love, has insoluble problems. We listen in our own poverty—not only our linguistic poverty, but also the poverty of being so new, of coming from somewhere else. We cannot respond in words, but only with our love and our prayers.

Language struggles

The intensity of Russian life and the demands of having to learn how to do every little thing were heightened by our acute language limitations. This was undoubtedly the single most exhausting factor in our life. Each task and each encounter meant trying to find the right words. Every night we fell exhausted into our beds. When we had guests and the conversation went on too long, Alma sometimes gave up the struggle to understand and fell asleep right at the table.

I did most of the speaking and interpreting, but Marie, with her Slavic background and, even more, her quality of deep listening, often understood more than I did. Alma considered herself fortunate if she managed to say hello and good-bye at the correct times, but much more important to our Russian friends was her wide smile, boundless hospitality, and readiness to help anyone with anything at any time.

Several people, including Inna and Tanya, volunteered to tutor Marie and Alma in Russian. The greatest obstacle to any real progress, however, was that our lives were so busy that neither of them had time to study.

That none of our friends except Alvina and Inna spoke English was ultimately to our advantage: we were forced to use whatever

---

* In the North women receive their pension when they reach fifty years of age and men, at age fifty-five. In other parts of Russia, the retirement ages are fifty-five and sixty.

vocabulary we had, supplemented by intuition and lots of shared laughter. Our friends were patient and encouraging as we slaughtered their beautiful language. We were grateful for those who had the gift of speaking simply and clearly in a way we could understand, and we marvelled at their ability to translate our garbled sentences into a Russian comprehensible to others.

We never knew for sure what was happening at any given moment. We didn't have a TV in those days, and we couldn't understand the kitchen radio that came with the apartment and broadcast the official government station. In the first days of October, while still living at the hotel, we had seen people huddled around the television and had understood that there was some kind of conflict in Moscow between Yeltsin and the Russian Parliament. Only later did we realize how serious the situation had been, and that a different outcome might have cut short the future of Madonna House in Russia.

The Catholic Parish of the Nativity

At the time of Jean and Marie's 1992 visit, Sunday Mass was being celebrated on the third floor of the building where our hotel was located. Now, a year later, the parish was meeting in a movie theatre, while awaiting the renovation of a fourth-floor room in a large, poorly-heated building on Gorky Street, less than fifteen minutes from our house. The move took place in November 1993, and our old people, most of them arthritic and short of breath, uncomplainingly scaled the four long flights of steep, uneven stairs to attend Mass.

We quickly realized that in Magadan, the word "church" did not denote a building but a community of faith, founded on and sustained by the sacraments. This parish community took us into its heart and became for us a never ending source of spiritual inspiration and support.

During these years, the Catholic Church in Russia, whose entire administrative structure had been wiped out during the Soviet era, was in the process of rebirth. In 1993 two bishops were consecrated and appointed apostolic administrators for European Russia and for Siberia and the Far East. Both were enormous territories. Everything had to be reconstructed. Since pre-revolutionary Catholics had worshipped in Latin, all the liturgical texts had to be translated into Russian. While experts laboured painstakingly over the wording, Fr.

Austin's translator, a student at the University of Magadan, translated the prayers from the English sacramentary, week by week, as best she could, for use at the Sunday Masses.

A wingless turkey

It was Marie's idea to schedule our official opening for December sixth, which was the feast of St. Nicholas, one of the most beloved saints in Russia. For our open house, Fr. Austin Mohrbacher offered us the frozen turkey he had just brought back from Anchorage. We roasted it on the evening of the fifth, and when we took the turkey from the oven, the aroma was so irresistible that we sliced off the wings and devoured them right then and there!

On the day of the celebration, we went to church for noon Mass and discovered that the liturgy had been rescheduled for *our* house that evening! Since we didn't know enough to do anything spontaneously, this required additional last-minute preparations.

In the afternoon friends began to bring food for the reception, which in Russia was simply called "tea." Young Kirill arrived ravenous from school, bit into a fish *pirozhok** and immediately spit it into his teacup, informing us that he was deathly allergic to fish. He told us not to worry; he would let us know if he felt sick!

By seven o'clock almost thirty people had gathered in the chapel. The children sat on the floor and the adults crowded behind them on chairs and stools. Fr. Austin was the last to arrive. We lit the Advent wreath, and he proceeded to celebrate a beautiful Mass with everyone joining in to sing—not the songs we had prepared, but those started by our obliging parish musicians!

After the liturgy, Fr. Austin blessed enough holy water so that everyone could take some home. As we processed through the apartment, he sprinkled every corner, looking as if he were enjoying himself. We finished in the living room before the icon of Our Lady of Kazan, singing "Rejoice, Virgin Mary," an Orthodox hymn that was part of our Madonna House repertoire.

Marie offered a few words of welcome: "Madonna House is the house of Our Lady, which means it is your house, too. We want you

---

* *Pirozhok* – the diminutive of *pirog*: meat, fish, vegetables, or fruit wrapped in dough and baked.

to come and visit, whenever you can. Come and pray. Come and rest in the hearts of the Lord and his Mother." She thanked everyone for their goodness and their help, and we distributed St. Nicholas Day gifts, explaining that each person was to pray for the one whose name appeared on the piece of paper he drew.

The food disappeared as fast as we set it out. The three of us were so busy that we never had a chance to eat and were glad we'd consumed the turkey wings the night before!

Halfway through the evening, Alvina came rushing into the kitchen, exclaiming, "Alexandra is dying on Miriam's bed!" Someone phoned the emergency medical service, and just as Fr. Austin was anointing the sick woman, three people in white coats entered the bedroom, having let themselves into the apartment. Alexandra survived and eventually walked home, escorted by two other guests. I was so busy in the living room that I didn't even know this was happening.

People began leaving around nine o'clock. Just as it seemed we might have time to pull ourselves—and the house—together, two more friends arrived, bearing a bouquet of huge chrysanthemums. We pulled out what was left of the food and visited with them. Soon the two women who had accompanied Alexandra returned, and it was eleven-thirty before this new gathering began to disperse.

Leaving the clean-up for the next morning, we collapsed into bed with a premonition that Marie's invitation—"This is the house of Our Lady, so it is the home of everyone"—was in danger of being taken quite literally.

Prayers for the dead

With each day the weak December sun sank lower towards the horizon. There was not a lot of snow, but the temperature went down to minus twenty-five Celsius, and the freezing crosswind from the two bays often chilled us to the bone. We learned to respect its ability to almost knock us off our feet as we rounded the corner of our apartment building. It was a challenge to stay upright on the icy sidewalks and streets. As we slipped and slid along, each of us took some hard spills, but we were grateful there were no real injuries.

Below us, in a one-room apartment on the first floor lived Margarita and her three companions: Tamara, Vasya, and Mitya.

Margarita had short grey hair, lively blue eyes, and broken teeth. We never knew at what hour of the day or night she would pop up to see us, but if she came early in the morning, it would inevitably be the one day we had planned to sleep in. Sometimes she came to borrow something; at other times to bring us a salted fish or a tasty vegetable dish. As we drank tea together, her wit and storytelling would keep us laughing.

On the morning of December sixteenth, Margarita came early to telephone the emergency service. The night before, while the others were away, Tamara had consumed two bottles of Korean vodka. Returning after midnight, Margarita found her passed out on the floor and put her to bed. By morning Tamara was dead.

We went down with Margarita, bringing holy water and a small book of Orthodox prayers. Tamara was lying on the bed, her face to the wall, with dried blood on her mouth and cheeks. As Alma said in all seriousness, she looked "very dead!" Marie blessed the body and the apartment with holy water, and I read the prayers for the deceased in Church Slavonic. Margarita, Mitya, and Vasya looked on silently, but with reverence. They were visibly shaken. Tamara had only been fifty-four.

For the next weeks we witnessed Margarita's determined efforts to beg money so that Tamara might be buried in an individual plot rather than in a common grave. "As if she was a dog," said Margarita indignantly. She succeeded, but just barely. After standing in the cold at the cemetery for several hours, clad in a thin coat and light boots, she came back with hypothermia. Marie and Alma were both nurses and worked for a long time to warm her.

Within three years, Margarita, Vasya, and Mitya were also dead from alcohol abuse.

A love that will never change—our first Christmas in Russia

I doubt if anyone in North America or Europe has ever experienced, as we did that year in Magadan, a Christmas so totally devoid of advertising glitter. After the Russian Revolution, religious feasts had been replaced by secular holidays. Traditions such as the Christmas tree, gift-giving, and family gatherings had been transferred to New Year's, which then became the most popular celebration of the year. Orthodox Christmas didn't fall until January sev-

enth in accordance with the Julian calendar and had only recently
been reinstated as a public holiday.

In 1993 the twenty-fifth of December fell on a Saturday, which
in Russia was an ordinary work and school day. Since Fr. Austin had
not scheduled Midnight Mass, we decided to invite some friends to
join us for a Christmas Eve prayer vigil and refreshments.

By five o'clock that afternoon, Marie was still baking Christmas
cookies. A friend—squeezed between the sink and the kitchen table—
was trying to wash dishes, and a ten-year-old was helping me copy
out Christmas carols in Russian. Soon there were more children,
more dishes, more noise— in short, loosely organized chaos.

Eight adults, five children, and three Madonna House staff workers eventually gathered in the chapel. On the altar, flanked by pine
branches and vigil lights in glowing green and red glass holders,
stood a beautiful Nativity carving by one of our Madonna House sisters. Our nervousness at leading a prayer service in a language none
of us spoke well was quickly dispelled by the loving support of our
friends, who led the five decades of the rosary, filled in the prayers
I'd left out, prayed the readings from the Vigil Mass, and joined in
a heartfelt Russian rendition of *Silent Night*. The spontaneous prayer
intentions embraced the whole world: believers and non-believers;
Catholics, Orthodox, and Protestants; our community, families,
friends, and enemies.

People were delighted by our simple Christmas decorations. In
the living room, the little artificial tree we had discovered in one of
the closets was decorated with four coloured glass balls, a few strands
of tinsel found with the tree, walnut shells wrapped in coloured foil
from a box of chocolates, and two or three ornaments given to us as
gifts. From cardboard and aluminum foil Marie had fashioned a silver star for the pinnacle of the tree. A crèche, icon prints, Christmas
cards, and brightly-coloured cloths completed the decorations. From
the corner of the room, called the "beautiful corner" in Russian, a
vigil lamp flickering softly before her, the icon of Our Lady of Kazan
watched over us all.

After our guests had departed and the three of us had sat down
to relax with a glass of wine, Lyuba, Fr. Austin's assistant, came to
pray in the chapel. She eventually joined us for tea and had just left
when Marina, another friend, appeared at the door, having seen the

Wayfarer's candle burning in our kitchen window. Late as it was, she knew she would be welcome. This was Marina's first Christmas as a Catholic.

On Christmas Day many regular parishioners were unable to leave their jobs to attend Mass, but other worshippers arrived, some of whom we had never seen before. Overflowing the seating capacity of the room, they stood along the walls and in the aisles. Nina, the choir director, was working, and her teen-aged choir girls were at their Saturday morning classes, but the congregation sang from their hearts all five verses of "Silent Night," and "How Great Thou Art" at the recessional. The kiss of peace went on and on, as people pushed through the crowded room to embrace each other. Fr. Austin baptized four children and three adults and then stood gazing upon his new parishioners with such paternal tenderness that it brought tears to our eyes.

There had been nothing in the streets to remind us that it was Christmas, but in that rented hall on the fourth floor of a commercial and office building, the coming of Christ was celebrated with a sincerity and depth of faith that surpassed anything we had ever experienced. The hopes, dreams, and future of every believer present were in the hands of the Saviour born to Mary in Bethlehem.

Most of the friends who came to celebrate with us that afternoon and evening, or who phoned to express their good wishes, were non-believers. One call was from the self-styled atheist who had so poignantly translated into Russian Catherine's book *My Russian Yesterdays*. Elbruss appeared at the door in a suit and tie, a white chrysanthemum in his hand, and joined us for tea. Ella Ostapenko was away in St. Petersburg, so we had invited Vasily and were only mildly surprised when he arrived with Dima, a non-believing Jew, and Dima's nominally Orthodox wife, Zhenia.

They had brought a bottle of Russian champagne and offered a toast "to the feast."

"To Christmas," Marie added quietly.

"To your beautiful faith," said Dima, "even though I don't share it myself."

The table conversation was not easy. Although the Soviet Union had ceased to exist, Vasily told us, they were all still Soviets. No one knew if the present freedoms would last, and daily life was becoming more and more precarious. We had just heard that in a town only five hundred kilometres north of Magadan, a power plant accident had left ten thousand people without heat or electricity in temperatures of minus fifty Celsius.

After our guests had left, Marie, Alma, and I struggled to find words for the impressions flooding our hearts. Again and again in Russia, we were to experience this mingling of joy and pain. But with the baptisms that morning, we had seen new shoots of spiritual life budding forth from the ruins of communism. Again and again, Fr. Austin had proclaimed, "Christ is born!" and the people had responded, "Glorify him!"

Jesus was born, he rose from the dead, and in this desolate city on the furthest edge of Russia, a tiny group of people had been given, through grace, the eyes to see his victory. We had been given the privilege of standing with them as they struggled to rebuild their lives on faith.

On Christmas Eve, Marina had said to us, "We Russians long for spiritual rest. Communism promised golden tomorrows, and they based their ideology on Christian values. Maybe that was why we went along with it and why, now that it has all collapsed, some of us turn so naturally to God. It's not teaching we hunger for. Everything around us is uncertain. No one knows what the future will bring. But to know God exists, that there is a love that will never change and that we can't lose, no matter what we do—*this* means everything to us!"

Renouncing Control

Along with fatigue from the relentless intensity of life and from the strain of trying to understand a new language and culture, one of the most difficult aspects of our new existence was its unremitting togetherness.

We were so different from one another! Marie had been raised in New York City by parents who had emigrated from Czechoslovakia. Alma had grown up on a farm and had been a Mennonite pastor before becoming a Catholic. I had just come from eight years of living in Paris. Our personalities, our ways of experiencing life, and our ways of relating were all different. This diversity of perspectives enriched our house diary and monthly newsletters, but living together twenty-four hours a day in what, for us, were very confining quarters was a considerable challenge.

Not to have a place where we could go regularly for a twenty-four hour poustinia was a genuine deprivation. When one has been making a weekly poustinia for many years, this becomes a way of life; a way of keeping one's heart before God and one's balance in community.

Regardless of whether or not we had a poustinia, we knew we would not survive in Magadan without prayer. Atonement for the evil perpetrated in this land was an integral part of our call here, and spiritual battle was ever-present in our lives, compounding and exacerbating our normal struggles. The city in which we lived had been built to serve a penal system designed to destroy the human person created in the image and likeness of God. In what once had been a Christian country, a sustained attempt had been made to eradicate God from the life and memory of its citizens. Satan had claimed this land as his own and would not easily relinquish it.

Difficult as it was to be without our own poustinia, we learned from the experience. It was an opportunity to lift up in prayer, to offer for others, a situation that was beyond our control. The lack of solitude became an invitation to identify with our Russian friends and their chronic lack of privacy. The absence of an escape hatch pushed us beyond what we considered to be our limits, since our own resources were insufficient for what God was asking of us.

When other options were exhausted, we threw ourselves on God's mercy—and he sustained us.

This was a Russian lesson we never finished learning.

The publication of Poustinia

To bring Catherine's words back to Russia was another important aspect of our apostolate. I had been asked by Jean to take responsibility in this area and, specifically, to work with Alvina on the translation and publication in Russian of Catherine's works.

When we came to Magadan, *Poustinia* was already at the regional publishing company. On October fourteenth, three weeks to the day after our arrival, Alvina telephoned to say we had forty-eight hours in which to check the final proofs before the book went to press! I raced over to her apartment where we worked until 2 A.M., broke off for a few hours of sleep, then worked some more. She read aloud from the Russian translation, and I followed along in English. Knowing that my Russian was totally inadequate for the task, I prayed desperately that God would show me the most important errors. We both chuckled at one ingeniously mistaken induction, inspired by Alvina's stay in Combermere: having translated literally the expression "chewing the fat," she wrote in a footnote: "A reference to the Madonna House custom of serving cracklings at afternoon tea!"

As we worked our way through the pages, I was moved to hear concepts that had become so much a part of our communal life expressed in the language in which they had traditionally been lived. Hearing *Poustinia* in Russian reminded me of reading the first lines of *Genesis* in Hebrew.

Few things happen on schedule in Russia, but we had no way of knowing what was behind the subsequent delays. As Alma said, "It's like rushing out of poustinia to help bring in the hay before it rains—and then it doesn't rain!" At one point, the director of the publishing house disappeared for over a week. We learned that he suffered from alcoholism and that the company itself was on the verge of bankruptcy.

The spiritual warfare surrounding this project was, for us, an indication of its significance. All we could do was to pray, and we prayed fervently.

On December 15, 1993, Marie wrote in our house diary:

Miriam and I accompanied Alvina to the publishers in the hope of finding out what was really going on. The director was back on the job, looking rather meek and sheepish and letting Tatiana, the editor, do the actual negotiations. It seems the old contract has expired, and a new one needs to be written. Miriam fielded some significant questions, and to make a long story short, more money is needed. The situation is very complicated, but inflation is the major factor. They said work could begin as soon as we make part of the payment, and that the book could be ready by the end of February. However, we have heard that kind of projection before! All things considered, we were satisfied with the meeting and feel there may be some hope. One advantage of the new contract is that we will be printing only five thousand copies, which seems infinitely more manageable than the ten thousand originally planned!

March 9, 1994 (Miriam writing)

This morning, Marie, Alma, Alvina, and I went to the publishing house, a twenty-minute walk across town, to receive the first copy of *Poustinia* in Russian! In English this is known as the "signal copy," and it seemed only right to present it to Alvina, whose initiative, enthusiasm, and skill had made the publication possible.

The first thousand copies have been completed, and the editor accompanied us to the printers to fetch as many packages as we could carry. She ended up arranging for someone there to give us a lift home with about three hundred copies. The driver refused to accept any money.

Fr. Austin has kindly offered us space in one of the fourth floor rooms to store the whole printing. We will soon begin mailing individual copies to friends in Russia and Europe, but the rest of the distribution will have to wait until we all return from holidays at the end of May.

The first person in Magadan to whom we sent a copy of *Poustinia* was the Orthodox bishop, Rastislav. As we wanted to introduce ourselves and to receive his blessing, we had been trying, without success, to reach him at his office to set up an appointment. Finally I thought to ask Lyuba, who gave me the bishop's home phone number. He answered my call on the first ring. Yes, he had received the book, he told me, and yes, he would be very happy to meet with us.

At this juncture, the bishop was still working out of a tiny office in the basement of the Orthodox church. Arriving a little early for our appointment, we were ushered into a little room to wait for Vladika,* as he was both addressed and referred to by the Orthodox faithful. About ten minutes later he entered, smiling, with apologies for having made us wait and for the shabbiness of the room. We greeted him simply in the Orthodox manner, holding out our cupped hands for his blessing and then kissing his ring.

We had known that the bishop was only thirty-two, but we were surprised by the quiet authority with which he moved. Small and slight, he had blue eyes, auburn hair pulled back and held by an elastic band, and a brownish-red beard. He had only been in Magadan since early December.

Thanking us for the book, he described it as "authentic Gospel spirituality" and said it would help many people. I managed to tell him who we were, who Catherine was, and that we had come to Magadan to love, serve, and pray; to listen and learn, and to walk with people, being to them as Simon of Cyrene. Vladika listened attentively—he seemed moved. After telling us he was glad we were in Magadan, he presented us each with newly-published booklets on Orthodox saints, gave us his blessing once again, and told us this would not be our last meeting.

To say that we were walking on air as we left would be the understatement of the year! We hardly spoke Russian, Vladika didn't speak English, but we had met spiritually.

The friendship and support of the librarians at the Pushkin Library was another gift from God. At their initiative, an official presentation of *Poustinia* was arranged for Easter Tuesday, April fifth, in the big library reception room. A floral exhibition had taken place there a few days earlier, and some of the flower baskets still remained. The librarians had made a display of Madonna House

---

* Vladika – literally, "Master" in Church Slavonic.

books, and we added a poster with photographs of Catherine and the Apostolate.

The gathering was small—about thirty people, many of whom we knew by face, if not by name, and also a number of our own friends. There were two radio journalists and two from the television stations. One of the TV journalists was our close friend Vasily, assisted by his wife, Ella.

The director of the library gave a short introduction in which she emphasized the unique quality of *Poustinia* and that we had chosen to publish it here in Magadan. She was convinced that the book's spiritual message was greatly needed at this time in Russia and that it would help many people. A librarian then introduced Alvina.

(Marie Javora writing)

As I sat and watched Alvina, I could not help but marvel at how much God had done in her soul and how he was now shining through her. Her face was radiant, really beautiful, as she recounted the story of how *Poustinia* had fallen into her hands. She also talked about Catherine, about her life in Russia and as a refugee, and about the founding of Madonna House.

Miriam spoke next, and if she was nervous, it wasn't at all apparent. She spoke of the gift we had received from Russia through Catherine and how happy we were to bring back to Russia what had been given to us. She explained how Catherine had realized that because the problems facing modern civilization had spiritual roots, the solutions had to be spiritual as well. She spoke of the poustinia of the heart as being the essence of poustinia.

When the three of us went on holidays at the end of April, I flew to Moscow to spend a month with Raia and Volodya. Now that I was actually living in Russia, how different everything seemed!

The Erokhins met me at the airport. While we waited for my luggage, I chattered away until I noticed them looking at me strangely.

"Am I talking too much?" I asked with some embarrassment.

Volodya burst out laughing. "You aren't talking too much; you are talking in *Russian!*"

One of the reasons I had wanted to come to Moscow had been to find contacts for the distribution of *Poustinia*. The channels that had existed before the fall of the Soviet Union were no longer operative, and I had no idea where to start. I felt like a babe in Toyland, but I kept asking the Holy Spirit for guidance.

One day I managed to reach Archbishop Kondrusiewicz by telephone, and to my surprise, he was able to see me that afternoon. I came away from the meeting with the addresses of all the Catholic parishes in European Russia and a suggestion that I contact Jean-François Thiry, the young Belgian director of an organization that distributed religious books throughout the country. This was exactly what I was looking for.

When I met Jean-François two days later, I could hardly believe my good fortune. His organization, the Library of the Spirit, was sponsored by the Catholic Church in European Russia and by Aid-to-the-Church-in-Need. He had a wide range of contacts among the Catholic parishes in the countries of the former Soviet Union, as well as some of the more open Orthodox parishes, and he offered books to them at half price. If we could arrange to ship *Poustinia* from Magadan to Moscow, Jean-François was more than willing to distribute it for us.

Orthodox Easter

A particular gift during this stay was the opportunity to celebrate Holy Week and Easter with the Orthodox Church. In Magadan, this was never feasible. Although we had originally hoped to attend Orthodox services from time to time, we discovered that it was physically and psychologically impossible to live two liturgical lives, each governed by a different calendar.

Raia and Volodya wanted to attend the Paschal Vigil in the town of Zvenigorod, about an hour and a half from Moscow by electric train. The ancient parish church, with frescos by Andrei Rublev, was now functioning, and Volodya knew the priest. As there was no return transportation until morning, we would be there all night.

Arriving at the Zvenigorod station a little before 10 P.M., we made our way leisurely past an eighteenth century church, now used as an administration centre, and past an old country estate. The twilight was fading as we found ourselves on the edge of a field. In the distance, we saw the church, perched on a hill.

"How long a walk will it be?" Raia wanted to know.

"Two hours," Volodya answered.

"Two hours!" we gasped in unison.

"Are you serious?" Raia asked. "A two-hour walk and then three hours standing at the liturgy?"

"I thought it would be a pilgrimage," he explained weakly.

Raia was silent and furious as we picked our way through the fields and bushes. There was nothing else to do, for the bus had long since departed by another route. Since it was growing dark and, not having expected a hike, I was wearing slippery dress pumps, I concentrated on not breaking my neck. Thank goodness, I still had my Magadan flashlight in my purse.

By the grace of God, we made it to the town. It seemed that most of the young people in Zvenigorod were also heading toward the church, many of them none too sober. As we climbed the stairs leading up the hill, a drunken man tumbled down smack into Volodya, and they fell together. Had not Volodya's knapsack, which was stuffed with food, cushioned his fall, he could have been seriously injured, and in her concern for him, Raia forgot she was angry. I was pushed against the railing and almost lost my own balance. We were all shaken and made our way as quickly as possible into the church.

I was not yet accustomed to Russian crowds. The church was small and solidly packed with people. Had I suffered from claustrophobia, I would have been hysterical; as it was, I was simply terrified. Volodya gripped Raia and me tightly by the arm and literally rammed a way through the crowd with his body, dragging us after him, to a side door that opened onto a narrow staircase leading to the choir loft. We positioned ourselves on the steps, where we had air to breathe and a view of the Royal Doors in the iconostasis.

Our refuge was more precarious than we realized. As we sat quietly, listening to the chant, a man with flaming red hair, peaked eyebrows, and wild eyes—obviously disturbed—rushed past, then turned to upbraid us in a loud voice for blocking the way. When the choir came piling down from the balcony for the procession with the cross, we had to move and once again found ourselves in the thick of the crowd, who by now were all holding lighted candles. I was certain there would be a fire and that anyone not burned to death would be trampled in the ensuing panic.

Volodya and Raia had an inspired idea. Instead of joining the procession around the outside of the church, we stashed our bags under a side table and positioned ourselves in such a way that when everyone came back indoors, we would be right in front of the iconostasis. As we breathed in and out, enjoying the respite and the Rublev frescos, we heard the first, soft strains of the Paschal chant:

> *O Christ our Saviour,*
> *The angels in heaven sing a hymn of praise to your Resurrection.*
> *As for us who dwell on earth,*
> *Make us worthy to glorify you with pure hearts.*

Louder and louder it swelled, and then, finally, came the long-awaited words, "*Christ is risen from the dead, trampling on death by death, and on those in the tombs, lavishing light!*"

The church filled up once more. People pressed around us, holding their candles. To my consternation, the line for confession* formed right next to us, adding to the pushing and shoving. I kept my eyes fixed on Volodya for security. I was more than a little nervous that I might faint. In such an atmosphere, who could pray?

What happened next was an absolutely new experience. It was not emotional, nor could it be explained as a crowd phenomenon. I found myself surrounded, caught up, and carried by the event we were celebrating, by the reality of the Resurrection made present by the liturgy. I was lifted on waves of singing that never ceased for two-and-a-half hours. Again and again the Easter verses burst forth, and the smiling priest emerged from the Royal Doors again and again to bless us with the three intertwined candles that represented the Holy Trinity, proclaiming the threefold "*Khristos voskrese!* Christ is risen!" followed by the resounding response, "*Voistinu voskrese!* Indeed he is risen!"

I followed the others to communion. Having gone to confession on Holy Thursday, and having just heard in Church Slavonic the fa-

---

* In Orthodox churches, confessions take place in the open church and continue during the liturgy.

miliar words of the Easter homily of St. John Chrysostom enjoining no one to go away hungry from this royal banquet, I had no doubt that I, despite being a Catholic, was also invited to the feast.

Afterwards—even after the two-hour hike and three hours of standing in the church—when it was all over and the congregation was filing out into the crisp night air, I had only one wish, one burning desire: that the liturgy would start all over again and never, never finish!

Acquaintances of Raia and Volodya invited us to a collation in the small parish house next door. We contributed our provisions, including *paska** and *koolitch*.** Others had also brought these traditional Easter desserts, and there were other foods as well, and wine, and of course, tea. Again and again we sang and proclaimed, "Christ is risen! Truly he is risen!"

It was almost 6 A.M. as we made our way in the early dawn to the bus that brought us to the train station for our return to Moscow. By nine we were home for our own breakfast of *koolitch* and *paska*, eggs and fruit, coffee and liqueur. We could hardly keep our heads up from fatigue, but none of us wanted the celebration to end.

Meeting Catherine in St. Petersburg

I could have basked in the Easter liturgy all week, but "Radiant Week," as the Easter octave is called in Russian, was the only interval into which Raia and I could sandwich a trip to St. Petersburg.

Fr. Georgy Friedman, a Russian Jewish Byzantine-rite Dominican, whose father had spent twenty years in the labour camps of Kolyma, and who had baptized Raia the previous summer, accompanied us to the apartment where Catherine's family had lived, only a ten-minute walk from the Hermitage Museum. I had no trouble picturing her in these streets, most of which seemed largely unchanged since the time of the Revolution.

Catherine had both talked and written about her life in St. Petersburg, where both her parents had been raised and where they had maintained a large apartment that occupied the third floor of

---

* Traditional Russian Easter dessert representing the Spotless Lamb and consisting of drained cottage cheese, butter, eggs, sugar, and raisins.

** A rich, sweet bread with spices, nuts, and candied fruit, baked in a tall metal can.

a building on the corner of Bolshaya Morskaya and Gorokhovaya Streets. Much of her childhood had been spent in the foreign countries to which her father's business had taken him, with summers at the family estate in Tambov. In 1910 the Kolyschkines returned to St. Petersburg, where thirteen-year-old Catherine enrolled at the Princess Obolensky School for Girls. Less than three years later, she married her debonair first cousin, Boris de Hueck.

The young couple moved to an apartment a few blocks away, on Gerlova Street. World War I found them both at the front: Boris as an engineer and Catherine as a nurse. When the Revolution broke out in February 1917, culminating in Lenin's seizure of power in October, the world Catherine had known gave way to one of danger and persistent hunger. Informed by a friend that their arrests were imminent, she and Boris had escaped to Finland.

As we approached the building where the Kolyschkine family had lived, Fr. Georgy told me that St. Petersburg entrances were notorious for their foul odours. This one smelled distinctly of urine. On the third floor were two apartments; we pressed the doorbell on the left. It was broken. We knocked. No answer. I was ready to try the other apartment when, to our amazement, we saw that the door was unlocked. This never happens in cities.

"Catherine opened it for us!" Raia whispered. Holding our breath, we went in.

The place was obviously a communal dwelling, cluttered and dingy. As we looked around, loudly clearing our throats to attract attention, a slovenly-looking young woman emerged from behind a half-closed door. Fr. Georgy explained that we knew someone who had lived here before the Revolution and would like to look around. The girl was unexpectedly obliging.

We could see where the original rooms, with the exception of the large kitchen, had been partitioned. Everything, of course, was rundown and shabby. I was too stunned to ask questions. The girl said that the original apartment had been divided in two; the other section was being remodelled, but since it was a holiday, no one was there.

As we left, all three of us were filled with awe. Fr. Georgy said, "If Madonna House ever comes to St. Petersburg, wouldn't it be wonderful if they could buy these same apartments?" A few days later, when Orthodox friends told us how moved they were to receive a copy of *Poustinia*, Raia mused, "It is as if St. Petersburg were welcoming Catherine."

The next day Raia and I went to the Smolensk cemetery, on the outskirts of the city, where the tomb of Blessed Ksenia of St. Petersburg is enclosed in a small chapel erected in her honour. Nearby stands the Church of Our Lady of Smolensk, which Ksenia helped to build by secretly carrying bricks in the night. Ksenia, who lived during the eighteenth century, had become a *yourodivyi*, a "fool for Christ," as a way of interceding for the soul of her deceased husband. Remembering Catherine's story of how, as a child, she had once set out alone on pilgrimage, I wondered if she might not have been going to this shrine, so beloved by the people of St. Petersburg.

After lighting candles before the icon of Blessed Ksenia, praying before her tomb, and circling the outside of the chapel three times, as prescribed by custom, Raia and I placed our petitions in a crack of the chapel wall. We then sat down to rest on a stone bench in the cemetery. Old women in kerchiefs strolled past. Raia drew my attention to one elderly woman dressed in black, whose severe elegance and erect bearing identified her as a traditional St Petersburg lady. Few of them were left, Raia explained.

The sun warmed the air and our faces. The trees were budding. Cats slipped among the tombs, and birds alighted here and there on the bushes. Branches rustled, and shadows moved among the gravestones.

I started to speak and suddenly found myself choked by tears. I felt Catherine's presence, as distinctly as if she had been standing behind me.

Adventures in book distribution

The next week I returned to Magadan. By now we had decided to buy another apartment to use as a poustinia. We had just begun looking around when we learned that Vanda, the owner of the one-room apartment next to us, was moving out. Although we had been hoping for two rooms, the possibility of having a place right next door was too good to turn down. The price was reasonable, and the owner, who soon became a friend, began steps to privatize it so that it could be sold.* To our amazement, the owner of the third apartment on our landing, the one which did have two rooms, told us that she too might be moving in the next year or so. Could this be a sign we were meant to have *three* apartments?

Meanwhile, we faced the challenge of getting several thousand copies of *Poustinia* to Moscow. The only mail service from Magadan was by air, and this was prohibitively expensive. One possibility, also expensive but far cheaper than mailing, was to send them by ship to Vladivostok and then by train across the continent. The books would have to be boxed and sewn into cloth bags according to specification. When Lyuba, our perennial consultant and by now our close friend, began to check into this, the complications were discouraging.

It was Alma who came up with the idea of renting space in someone's container. "Isn't this how everyone moves things from Magadan?" she asked rhetorically.

Walking home from church one day, I ran into a woman named Anna, who lived just a few doors away from us, and whom Alma and I had met a few weeks earlier. Anna was moving to a town 108 kilometres from Moscow, and when she mentioned that she was expecting her container to arrive any day, I popped the question: would she be willing to sell us space in her container to ship our books? Her answer was affirmative.

The next step was to find out if Jean-François at the Library of the Spirit was willing to travel a hundred kilometres to pick up the books. For us, this arrangement would be cheaper, faster, and simpler than shipping. When I finally reached him by phone, Jean-François gulped once and then—to our amazement, joy, and infinite gratitude—agreed to do whatever was needed. He was familiar enough with Russian conditions to know that one had to make unusual efforts to accomplish seemingly ordinary ventures, and he continually went the extra mile.**

---

* In the USSR, all property was owned by the state. After the break-up of the Soviet Union, occupants had the option of either continuing to live as before or to privatize their apartments, which gave them the right to sell or otherwise dispose of them as they wished.
** In the years that followed, Jean-François continued to help us distribute our books. In 1999 the Library of the Spirit published the first Russian edition of *Fragments of My Life* under the title *Tales of a Russian Strannik*.

The following day, as Marie and I were preparing to go over in the drizzling rain to finalize arrangements with Anna, we glanced out the kitchen window and saw that among the amassed boxes we'd noticed earlier in front of her apartment building entrance, there were now pieces of furniture. Quickly putting two and two together, we deduced that the container parked before the building belonged to Anna, and it was being loaded *now*! We raced over.

No problem, Anna assured us. It would take her about three hours to load, and we had all that time to get our books ready. She said they would drive the container to the church building and load our boxes from there.

All that time! Within minutes, we had collected every bit of tape and string, scissors, plastic bags, and the few boxes we had in the apartment. We roused Alma, who had slept late in anticipation of a day off. By now it was raining profusely. On the main street, Proletarskaya, we hailed a passing car* to take us to Fr. Austin's to get the key for the rooms where the books were stored.

Once there, we sprang into action. Alma went out in search of more cardboard boxes, Marie started packing books into the boxes at hand, and I marked the boxes as they were filled. Soon Lyuba joined us. Our friend Nadia and a ten-year-old student from the choir school appeared and began hauling the boxes down the four long flights of stairs. At one point, I returned to where the container was being loaded to see how much space would be available and was told not to worry; there would be room for as many books as we could pack.

The truck with the container arrived, and Anna herself began to help us cart the books downstairs and onto the container. She was carrying boxes twice as large and heavy as those we ourselves could manage. We had bagged and boxed about two thousand copies when Marie finally said, "That's the end. I can't pack one more book!"

When the boxes had all been loaded into the container, I negotiated the price with Anna. Off they drove, and a little less than half

---

* There was not yet a taxi service in Magadan, but most drivers were happy to make a little extra money by taking passengers to points within the city.

our total printing was on its way across the Russian continent, sandwiched between Anna's bed linens, pots and pans, and furniture.

Meanwhile, another avenue of distribution had opened up. The Catholic parish in Vladivostok had an extensive outreach program, and the layman to whom I spoke on the phone was willing to distribute *Poustinia* to those on their mailing list. The books could be shipped to them as freight. Lyuba directed us to the office that made shipping crates. When the crates were ready, two of our librarian friends offered to go with me in the library minibus to pick them up at the workshop outside the city.

What a sight we were! One librarian in high heels, the other in a silk suit, and me, picking our way among the debris and rusting machine parts, trying to find the right entrance and the right crates. The workers helped us squeeze the five thirty-six kilogram wooden boxes into the aisle of the minibus, where we stood them on end with the heavy covers balanced on top. As the bus bumped and lurched along the dirt road to the highway, the three of us supported the crates and covers with our bodies to keep them from smashing into the windows.

How were we to get these heavy boxes up to our second-floor apartment? When we pulled up to our building, the driver and the librarians somehow managed to get them off the bus and on to the street. The driver, patently unenthusiastic about the whole business, drove off without further ado. Just then a macho-looking stranger disembarked from a jeep, and I asked him to help. He took a crate under each arm, deposited them on the landing in front of our door, and disappeared upstairs. At that moment Marie came out and commandeered a man who was coming toward us. He introduced himself as a neighbour we hadn't met and willingly lent a hand.

Pushing chairs and tables to the side, we made space for the crates on the living room floor, where they remained for the next week. Because the crates were built of unseasoned wood, with holes and spaces between the boards, we lined them with sheets of thick plastic to protect the books from water and dust. After Sunday Mass a long line of parishioners helped relay twenty-five hundred copies of *Poustinia* down from the fourth-floor storage room and onto a farm truck belonging to one of the parishioners. Another team of friends unloaded them at our apartment.

The next day I began packing them into the crates. Someone told us where to buy the two hundred nails needed to secure the crate covers, and our neighbour Slava came on two successive evenings to hammer down the lids.

The final step was to take the crates to the shipping yard by the seaport. On the designated morning, Lyuba arrived with an acquaintance who owned a truck. Two other men had been hired to carry and load the crates, each of which now weighed one hundred and thirty kilos. Lyuba and I rode to the port in the back of the truck. The dark, airless, bumpy ride reminded us both of the conditions under which political prisoners had once been transported.

It was a day of miracles.

At the shipping yard, we found ourselves in a sea of metal containers, facing a few rundown buildings. A lift drove up to the back of our truck, onto which our driver singlehandedly unloaded the heavy crates. These were driven over to the scales and weighed: six hundred and fifty kilos. The man weighing them informed us that the limit was five hundred kilos, above which the contents were supposed to be shipped by container. Lyuba said nothing, her face expressionless. I held my breath while the man wrote on the form, "Five hundred."

That was our first miracle.

The next moment a second miracle loomed before me, a broad smile on his face. I recognized Vitaly, the driver of the truck that had taken the container with our Moscow-bound books. He had gone out of his way to help us that day, and now we learned that he worked at the shipping yard. Even Lyuba hadn't realized the extent to which this was a man's world, and seeing the volume of traffic, she was quickly reaching the conclusion that we would never get the documents formulated that day without a connection. Enter Vitaly.

As we waited in the crowded shipping office, Lyuba, alert as always, noticed that all the transactions were accompanied by winks and meaningful glances. Vitaly had disappeared. Now Lyuba herself kept disappearing without an explanation. Only when Vitaly returned and we followed him out into the hall, where Lyuba began counting out money, did I surmise that he had made a private agreement with one of the clerks to take care of our papers. After ten months in Magadan, I knew better than to ask questions. Eventually we left the transaction to him and went for lunch in the big, empty cafeteria next door.

At 1 P.M. Lyuba's name was called. We jumped up and followed the clerk out into the yard to where our crates were stacked, unprotected, in the pouring rain. I prayed that the plastic inside had been well-sealed. The clerk informed us that the address, which I had so neatly written with a thick waterproof marking pen, was incorrect; the crates were not going to Vladivostok itself, but to a railroad shipping station. This now had to be marked on all six surfaces of all five crates, including the sides that were hidden from view by the crates above and below them. We were also supposed to write out names in full, without using initials.

Lyuba worked her magic to obtain some thin black paint, a stubby brush with bristles all clotted together, and a grimy rag. She insisted on doing all the readdressing herself, while I tried to shield her from the rain with my umbrella. But how were we to move the crates so that she could write the address on the undersides? The first worker to whom she appealed for help refused.

Miracle Number Three: the young man who had been directing incoming traffic was going on his break, and he graciously lifted, slid, and turned the crates for us, one by one.

The whole job took us two hours.

Back at the shipping office, I signed the papers and paid the shipping fees. After five-and-a half hours at the shipyard, we were finally finished.

The final challenge was to get back to town. The bus service was sporadic, and we were too cold and wet and tired to even think of walking. Lyuba, who had been straining, craning, and half the time literally writing upside down, was exhausted and soaked to the skin. Slipping some roubles to the old man who had lent us the paint, we left the shipyard and promptly spotted a van, parked but with its engine running, just down the road. The driver was going downtown and agreed to take us as far as his destination—right next door to the church office! This was the final miracle of this memorable day.

Fr. Michael

Our first Magadan summer continued with berry-picking and mushroom-gathering expeditions, hikes, and the frequent cleaning of fresh salmon, which was in such abundance. We bought Vanda's apartment and gently prodded her to start repainting the kitchen and bathroom as she had promised. Two new friends used the rolls of orange-patterned wallpaper we had found in a closet to redo the hall and main room. It was an innovation in poustinia décor, but we felt justified in using what God had provided.

In early September, the apartment was ready for use. We each began making weekly poustinias with renewed appreciation and gratitude for the gift of this privileged time with God.

On September fourteenth, the feast of the Exaltation of the Cross, we celebrated the first anniversary of the foundation of Madonna House in Magadan. The following day Fr. Michael Shields, a forty-four-year-old priest from the diocese of Anchorage, arrived to dedicate his life to "praying in the camps."

Tall and athletic, Fr. Michael had curly black hair and a full beard, smiling dark eyes, and a ready laugh. His grey habit, which he had designed himself, had a large red heart and cross emblazoned on the scapular. While remaining a diocesan priest, he wore it as a sign of monastic dedication in the spirit of Charles de Foucauld.

Having been submerged in parish responsibilities for thirteen years, Fr. Michael could hardly believe his good fortune in being able to spend his first eight months in Magadan studying Russian and praying. Each day he would concelebrate with Fr. Austin at the noon Mass, frequently returning with us for lunch and an hour alone in our chapel before the Blessed Sacrament. He was with us often, exuding vitality, an exuberant love of God, and a deep commitment to prayer.

Fr. Michael regarded community as essential to the Christian life, and he envisioned the formation of a small fraternity of priests dedicated to the spirituality of Charles de Foucauld and to Russia.* He had read Catherine's books and had been making weekly poustinias for several years.

Quite soon after his arrival, Fr. Michael began celebrating Mass in our chapel at 8 A.M. each Saturday morning in memory of those

---

* The foundation of the Little Brothers of the Heart of Jesus and the fulfillment of this dream began in 1996 with the arrival of Fr. David Means, also of the Anchorage archdiocese. His presence and gifts, which were complementary to Fr. Michael's, helped stabilize the parish.

who had died in the camps. Because of the early hour, on a day
when people could sleep in, only a few would join us, never more
than two or three. The same people continued to come fairly regularly over a period of time, feeling a particular call to pray with us.
After the liturgy, everyone shared a simple breakfast.

As always, we spoke Russian, translating for those who had trouble understanding. Fr. Michael suffered acutely from his poor command of the language, and since he was a priest, called to preach and
minister to the people of Magadan, his need was even more urgent
than ours. From the very onset, he celebrated the liturgy in Russian,
asking a native speaker to proclaim the Gospel until he could read it
fluently enough that his efforts would not be a distraction. When he
began preaching at the Sunday Masses, alternating with Fr. Austin,
he would write a simple homily in English for Alvina to translate and
then spend hours practicing until he could deliver it smoothly. For a
naturally-gifted preacher, this was a real frustration, but the spiritual
fruits were evident. The cumbersome process resulted in a powerful
simplicity of expression, and the inability to speak and relate easily
became a safeguard against relying on his natural talents. Language
handicaps had the advantage of keeping us all dependent on the
Lord and on the help of our friends.

Parishioners were encouraging and appreciative, responding to
his warmth and his desire to serve them not only spiritually, but in
practical ways as well. They felt close to him, just as they felt close
to us. The priesthood was Fr. Michael's deepest identity, eclipsing
any linguistic limitation. Over the years, he became more and more
profoundly a spiritual father to his parishioners.

A dissenting opinion

As much as I hated to admit it, and unlike practically everyone
else around me, I didn't care that much for Fr. Michael. Not at the
beginning.

First of all, he was around *a lot*. I was more introverted than either
Alma or Marie and found it more difficult to adapt to the Russian
hospitality that had no boundaries. Welcoming many people at once
left me depleted and exhausted. I craved solitude or, at the very least,
being alone with my sisters. Easy as Fr. Michael was to be with, his
frequent presence was for me a constraint.

I also found him loud and very American. In France, where I had lived for ten years, one of the highest accolades for a foreigner was to be told he was "discreet," meaning that he fit smoothly into the cultural landscape. Russians, on the contrary, never expected foreigners to be anything but different, and at that time, Westerners were still an intriguing novelty. Even so, every time Alma, Marie, and I left the house together, I cringed at our conspicuousness. Not only our clothes, but our smiles, the way we looked around as we walked down the street, the way we looked directly at the people we passed, and, of course, our English speech identified us as Americans. When Fr. Michael was with us, the effect was heightened. In his grey habit with its bright red emblem, he immediately drew stares.

His exuberance wearied me. It was all very well for him to wax eloquently about the joy of suffering out of love for Christ, I thought irritably, but we'd been trying to live it out a lot longer than he had!

"Throwing in my lot"

By January 1995 Marie, Alma, and I found ourselves drained from the Christmas season, the roller-coaster of daily life, and the spiritual oppression in the city. I found the differences between us almost insurmountable. Marie insisted that without unity we would not be able to withstand the spiritual pressures, but I felt I was at an impasse.

During my years in poustinia houses, I had learned, through much struggle, to rely on God, rather than others, for the fulfillment of my own emotional needs. As the director of our house in Paris, I had had to stand in aloneness and turn to God for personal support and guidance. My sense of self had been strengthened, and it seemed I had grown in emotional maturity.

Why, then, was I feeling so isolated in this new setting, this new configuration of people? Had my heart shrivelled? What had gone wrong?

Marie suggested that the loneliness I was experiencing might be of my own making, a consequence of the emotional detachment I had cultivated during my Paris years. Suddenly I heard God saying in my heart that my call now was to die to the self I had so painfully acquired, to not stand apart, but to "throw in my lot" with Marie and Alma.

The thought terrified me. Through tears I could barely control, I told Marie, "I feel as if I carry a whole world inside myself. It's a rich world, and I don't want to let go of it, but I hear God asking me not to cling to anything. It's my wealth—and he is calling me to become poor."

This stunned even Marie. "I wouldn't want to be in your shoes right now!" was all she could find to say.

I longed to forget the whole conversation. My stomach lurched each time I thought about it. Worst of all, I didn't know what, concretely, I was supposed to do.

"I don't understand," I kept telling God.

Praying before the icon of the Saviour, I felt myself held in his grave, compassionate gaze. *Miriam,* he seemed to be saying, *you will never understand with your mind. I am trying to reach your heart.*

Toward the end of March, Alma left to spend a few months in Canada. The pace never slackened, and by Easter Friday, the day of Marie's departure for the Directors' Meetings, the two of us were literally sick with fatigue.

Her flight was scheduled for late afternoon, and there was a possibility we might have a little time alone together before she left. Shortly before noon, we headed for the parish chapel on Gorky Street, where we joined the little group of weekday communicants outside the fourth-floor room, waiting for Fr. Michael to come for Mass. When Fr. Michael arrived, however, he discovered he had locked the chapel keys in his apartment. Rather than wait for someone to fetch them, he thought it would be simpler if we all adjourned to Madonna House and celebrated Mass in our chapel.

That's all we needed, I thought resentfully. Now we have to improvise a post-liturgy lunch for seven more people!

Back at the house, Marie and I quickly set up the altar. I was mentally trying to organize the meal. In response to a suggestion from Marie, I had bought a package of sausages and boiled a pot of potatoes in order to have some extra food on hand. She must have had a premonition, I thought. Darn it all, anyways; couldn't Fr. Michael be more organized?

As the Mass went on, I began to repent of my reaction. What was the point of being so constantly irritated and angry? This was Russia, and if I wanted to be here, I would have to take life on its own terms.

I will accept the chaos of this life, I told God silently.

It was a pure act of faith.

Raia in Magadan

Marie was planning to spend a few months in Washington D.C. after the meetings, resting and studying Russian. Alma would be back at the beginning of June, and soon afterwards Beth Holmes, another staff worker, would join us to lend a hand.

During this time, I would be in charge. In faith, I had to believe that since I had been asked to exercise this responsibility, God would give me the graces I needed. On a human level, however, I was only too aware of Marie's special charism for directing the house, and of my own deficiencies.

Raia came from Moscow to be with me in May, pending Alma's return. Insisting that she had not come as a guest, but to live our life and to help me, she did everything from cleaning the apartment in record time to marking the accents in our Russian prayer books so that we could pronounce the words properly. With warmth and sensitivity, she welcomed those who came to the house.

How much I learned from having a Russian at my side! For instance, she taught me not to ask politely, "Would you like to stay for supper?" but to insist on it. I learned never to hand anything through a doorway and not to sweep a floor when a departing guest has embarked on a plane but has not yet reached his destination—two deeply-engrained Russian superstitions. I learned the Russian way to make a bed and how to serve a meal properly. Raia paid us the ultimate compliment when she observed one day, "Madonna House receives people with Russian hospitality!"

Raia had no prejudice against Catholicism. Her Orthodox faith had been moulded by Fr. Men, and visits to Paris and Taizé had familiarized her with the Catholic Church and other Christian confessions. In Magadan, however, she experienced Catholicism from another perspective. Although some of our parishioners were Polish, Ukrainian, or Catholics from the Baltic countries, the majority were

ethnic Russians. Both Fr. Austin and Fr. Michael envisioned a Russian
Catholicism that did not require its adherents to adapt a foreign cul-
ture, but which was enriched by elements of Orthodox spirituality.
However, the parish was still its infancy, and the whole Catholic
Church in Russia was in the beginning stages of reconstruction.

Several nights before Raia left, I listened to her speaking with
some of our friends about Russian Orthodoxy. Her voice resonat-
ed with a love and a passion I'd never heard before. She spoke of
the stumbling blocks new churchgoers encountered—the irritating
babushkas who tell everyone what to do, the unfamiliar Church
Slavonic, the discipline of the fasts. She explained that these were
things to be moved through until one reached the living heart of
Orthodox faith. After that, she said, what at first seem like hindranc-
es to faith become supports to its practice.

I had the impression that here in Magadan Raia had finally discovered her religious identity. For the first time in her life, she realized the seriousness of the schism between East and West, the rend-
ing of the Body of Christ. "If it is so unbearable for me," she said,
"what must it be like for God?"

The day before she was to return to Moscow, a stream of people
came to the apartment to say goodbye. Some she had been drawn
to from the beginning; others she had had a harder time relating
to. When we finally closed the door late that evening, Raia was
radiant.

"Miriam, thank you!" she exclaimed. "You don't know what
Madonna House and Magadan have given me. I think I've learned
to see people as you see them—simply as they are. You've helped me
to open my heart again. You've shown me how to love."

A new conversion

Shortly after Raia's departure, Alma returned from Anchorage.
A week later, Beth arrived. To her delight, we began calling her Liza,
the Russian diminutive for Elizabeth.

In the months that followed, I was surprised to find in Fr. Michael
a source of both personal and spiritual support. He was readily available, non-judgmental, and I could turn to him to talk out ideas and
problems. I grew to appreciate his lucid mind, keen observation and
understanding of different personalities. I was also beginning to real-

ize that what I'd taken to be a romantic and somewhat flamboyant
spirituality had been won at a hard cost. I envied his delight in the
"little ones"—the poor and the marginal—who flocked to our house
and whom I often found so hard to accept. Most of all, I recognized
in his relationship with the Lord and Our Lady the passion and intimacy I was beginning to long for.

Fr. Austin was absent quite a bit that summer. When escalating
health problems made it necessary for him to return permanently
to North America, it was heartbreaking both for him and for the
parishioners to whom he had revealed the face of a loving God. Fr.
Michael became the acting pastor.

Alvina had finished translating Catherine's book *Soul of My Soul*,
and as a title for the Russian edition, she suggested "On the Heart
of Christ." I loved it. It evoked the image of St. John the Beloved,
as the Orthodox called him, leaning on the Lord's breast at the Last
Supper and feeling the heartbeats of divine love. For this reason, and
because of the yearning in my own soul, the feast of the Sacred Heart
held a particular intensity for me that year.

The celebration fell on a Saturday, and three of our friends
joined us for Mass in our chapel, followed by breakfast. As neither
Fr. Michael nor Alma could really converse in Russian, and Liza
could not speak at all, I always found myself walking a fine line between facilitating the conversation in a way that included everyone,
and dominating it. This time I got carried away. I knew I needed to
repent.

When I went to confession, Fr. Michael said that God was calling me to humility as a key to exercising responsibility. "Humility is
what wins trust," he said. God was not calling me to be strong, but
to be a servant.

His words were like cool water on the parched earth of my
heart. I was surprised at the gratitude that choked me. It wasn't the
first time I had felt in confession that he was responding to an even
deeper need than I was aware of. A door opened in my heart, and it
seemed as if the Lord were standing on the other side of the threshold, beckoning me to himself.

In my poustinia journal I wrote:

How strange to realize the extent to which I've lost the habit of trusting even a priest with my deepest heart! It is frightening now to put my soul in someone's hands and to let myself be led.

Why, how, did my heart turn to stone? What happened to me, that I have become so unable to open myself to others? Now I understand what Marie was praying for so intensely last winter. The challenge to "throw in my lot" touched something so deep that the pain and fear almost overwhelmed me, but I see now that it was the fear of surrender. I hadn't realized that the surrender is to *God,* and it takes place in a relationship of love.

For the past five years or so, my relationship with God has felt lifeless, like a marriage that still has moments when the flame is rekindled, but which has ceased to grow. Now something is stirring again. From the moment I first touched Russia, a passion I didn't even know I possessed was awakened in my heart. That's what this country evokes—not emotion, but passion! I now understand that the true object of that passion is Christ.

I began seeing Fr. Michael weekly. I found I could be direct with him, exposing what was in my heart without fear of what he would think. I told him that I had no trouble believing God loved me, probably because my own father had been so loving. I had my wounds, but I didn't think God was calling me to focus on them. The deepest desire of my heart was not to receive love but to give it, and the ultimate expression of love was self-giving. I'd seen what real love looked like in my sisters and in our Russian friends, and I was becoming painfully aware of my own lack of generosity and of my rejection of the poor. I wanted to touch Christ in a deeper way. I wanted to learn to love—and I needed help.

Fr. Michael replied that it wasn't a matter of emotional wounding, but of deep spiritual brokenness. To really know Christ I had to touch the crucified Lord, first in my own heart and then in the hearts of others, and especially in the little ones and those who suffered. Did I have the courage to take that journey inward?

At first I drew back. I had always been afraid that if I offered God everything, he would take me at my word. I'd never been able to freely pray Charles de Foucauld's "Prayer of Abandonment." To surrender myself "without reserve" was surely courting disaster!

I wanted to be certain Fr. Michael understood that I was *not* asking to become a victim soul. He reassured me that God had a path for each of us, a path of love. "He isn't asking you to fall apart. He is asking you to 'unlearn' who you are, to lay aside your certainties and definitions and ways of coping and understanding. But the road leads to the cross. Is that what you want?"

How could I say no? My rationalizations, my fears and excuses, and all my bids for affirmation and praise had proven sterile. I didn't want to play games any longer.

Fr. Michael emphasized that this was not a self-fulfillment program. We don't just eradicate these defects and start living a life free from sin. Rather, we learn that all we have to stand on is God's mercy.

We talked of the reality of sin and the need for constant repentance. "Sin is like a troika driven by pride," he said, quoting one of the Eastern Fathers. "The three horses are arrogance, judgment, and boasting. We need to replace pride by humility and the horses by purity of heart, mercy, and self-abasement."

To consciously place myself below others, as he suggested, didn't make sense to me. I thought it meant not placing myself higher and not rejecting or judging anyone, but Fr. Michael explained that it was a position of the heart, not of the mind. The Pharisee's sin against the Publican consisted in drawing comparisons. The only way out of this regrettable human tendency was to deliberately place oneself lower.

I heard this as a call to repent of my pride and arrogance and of my need to control. "When your heart is pure," Fr. Michael said, "you neither dominate others nor can you be dominated."

Once, when I knew Fr. Michael was preoccupied with a painful pastoral situation, I said apologetically, "I'm sorry to be talking about myself at a time like this."

"Miriam," he said, "It's exactly the opposite. What happens in the heart is what really matters."

This was almost a new language for me, and one I very much
needed to learn. For years I had turned away from those elements of
Catholic spirituality that displeased or threatened me. In the same
vein, I had preferred not to think too much about "Pain is the kiss
of Christ" and similar aspects of Catherine's teaching. Now, as new
tendrils of life began to unfurl in my heart, I realized how desperate
my situation had become. The clock had struck twelve: my spiritual
carriage was about to turn into a rotten pumpkin and the human
gifts that had hitherto sustained me—to dust. My only real choice
was between death and life through the acceptance of the cross.

This was the beginning of a new conversion. It was difficult,
draining, and exhausting. I needed to re-pattern a lifetime of habits.
"I am just taking baby steps," I wrote to Jean,

> but there is no other way for me now. I can hardly believe
> what God is doing—this is the kind of spiritual adventure
> Catherine used to speak about, and I feel a new closeness
> to her.

One day in early September, after a confession that had been
deeply healing, but which had left me feeling exposed and vulnerable, I took a shortcut home across an open area, carefully picking
my way among broken glass, rocks, scraps of metal, and pieces of
wood. Suddenly I stopped and looked up. The sky was a translu-
cent, autumnal blue, the air was crisp, and the sun streamed down
on my face. It was as if my whole being, including my femininity, lay
open to the Lord, and the unbounded warmth of his love radiated
into every pore of my skin. I was inundated with happiness.

I meet a staretz*

By now Marie had returned, and I was preparing for my holidays. I planned to spend some time in Moscow and then to visit an
Orthodox community in Latvia with which we had been in touch.

Archimandrite Viktor Mamontov was a Russian Orthodox priest
living in the town of Karsava, not far from the Latvian-Russian border. He and his lay co-worker, Alla, had learned of Madonna House

---

* In Russian tradition, a spiritual elder, who transmits his knowledge of God by
word and example.

in 1993 from a mutual friend, who told them about our foundation in Magadan. We began corresponding, and when we sent them copies of the Russian translation of *Poustinia*, Fr. Viktor passed them to his spiritual children. Soon we were receiving letters and requests for more books from Latvia, Russia, and Ukraine.

Born in 1938, Fr. Viktor grew up on the Sakhalin peninsula—a totally atheistic province, without churches or priests—on the far eastern coast of Russia. His father, an army officer, had been killed in World War II. In 1971 Fr. Viktor was baptized in Moscow, where he was teaching Russian literature at Moscow State University. His godmother was the sister of the great Russian poetess Maria Tsvetayeva, on whom he had written his doctoral thesis. He entered a Ukrainian monastery, but was forced to leave during the religious crackdown preceding the 1980 Moscow Olympics. For someone with a doctorate to enter the monastic life belied the official contention that religion was strictly the affair of superstitious old women.

Advised to go to Latvia, where things were quieter, he received the monastic tonsure in 1982, was ordained to the priesthood, and assigned a small parish not far from Riga. When the stream of students and young people coming to him attracted the attention of the KGB, Fr. Viktor's bishop sent him to the country parish of Karsava, hidden in the backwoods of eastern Latvia. Even there, people came to him from all parts of the Soviet Union. After the break-up of the USSR, when new borders and visa requirements made travel more complicated and more expensive, his spiritual children continued to seek him out, always with great delight and anticipation.

Among those who came to be near Fr. Viktor and help him in his work were Alla, formerly a professor of French at the University of Kiev; Anastasia, a Lithuanian, who cared for the church and sang with Alla at all the services; and eighty-year-old Serafima from St. Petersburg, who cooked for the parish and sold candles at the liturgies. Fr. Viktor claimed that when only the three of them were at the services, Serafima sold candles to the angels!

I fell in love with Karsava, a village with five thousand inhabitants, rows of one-story houses, and storks' nests in the trees. As Fr. Viktor was busy with visitors when I arrived, I didn't meet him until vespers that evening. It was December and already dark. With the snow crunching under our feet and the pungent scent of wood-burn-

ing stoves filling the winter air, Alla and I walked the short distance
from her house, where I was staying, to the church. Framed by tall
pines, light shining through the cupola, it reminded me a bit of Our
Lady of the Woods Chapel in Combermere.

Once inside, it took me a few minutes to adjust to the dimness.
Lampadas illuminated the faces of the icons, and a single lamp was
provided for the choir. Alla invited me to sit with her and Anastasia
so that I might follow the prayer book and sing along with them as I
could. First, however, they pushed me down beside the wood stove
so that I could warm up.

Just before the service, Fr. Viktor emerged from behind the
iconostasis, a slight figure even in his vestments. He was only fifty-
eight, but with his lined face and flowing white hair and beard, he appeared closer to seventy. I rose and went to him, cupping my hands
for his blessing, then kissing his hand in the Orthodox manner. This
was not a natural gesture for Catholics, but with him it felt instinctive. He took my hands in his, and as I looked up into his face, so full
of kindness, my heart leapt. He said to me, "It will be hard for you
with us, but your soul will rejoice."

I saw a good deal of Fr. Viktor that week. At the liturgies and
the communal meals following them, I was always touched by his
attentiveness. Whenever I was with him, I found myself wanting to
smile with all my being or to weep with all my heart.

Although I was a Catholic, it was taken for granted that I would
receive communion.

The length of the services and the lack of sleep were physically
draining. The evening of my arrival, two catechists from Moscow
gave a Scripture class to the community after vespers, followed by
a question-and-answer period that went on until midnight. Lauds
the next morning began at six, followed by the small hours, confessions, and the two-hour Divine Liturgy. I had thought Alla was
joking when she told me the liturgy finished at 11 A.M., but this was
a conservative estimate: one liturgy I attended was followed by a
funeral and another by a prayer service for the deceased. All this
took place on an empty stomach, since in the Orthodox Church,
those receiving Holy Communion had to fast from food and drink
after midnight.

No wonder Fr. Viktor looked so much older than his age, I thought. Alla told me he continued to observe the strict monastic rubrics, rising during the night to pray. Now that the pre-Christmas fast had begun, he hardly seemed to eat at all, but he was always putting food on my plate and saying with a smile, "You must eat; you are not used to fasting as we do."

As the week progressed, as I ate, slept, visited, and prayed, I realized I was participating in an integrated Orthodox lifestyle, lived simply but profoundly. I asked many questions and came to appreciate in a new way the unifying power of a life of faith. It reminded me of what I had experienced when I first came to Madonna House. I could almost feel my heart opening under what Fr. Michael would have described as "the pressure of grace."

Prayer accompanied everything we did. Alla and I went several times for lunch at the little house where Fr. Viktor lived with his sister, brother-in-law, an enormous German shepherd, and eight cats. The cats occupied every free surface in the kitchen, eating, sleeping, grooming themselves and each other. We prayed before and after each meal. When we entered Fr. Viktor's little office, crowded with books and papers, we would first turn to the icons in the corner and pray again before we began talking. One day when I had a bad headache, probably from lack of sleep, he anointed me. The headache passed, but the following day my back went out! Fr. Viktor assured me that these trials were to be expected since I was receiving such spiritual blessings.

He was quite interested in Catherine and in Madonna House, of which he already seemed to have an instinctive understanding. He and Alla spoke of their desire to build a poustinia. He called it *POUstinka*, meaning "little poustinia," with the accent on the first syllable. They studied my photographs of the Combermere poustinias and even wanted to know the measurements.

At the close of the Sunday liturgy, on the last day of my visit, Fr. Viktor called me to stand next to him in front of the iconostasis and introduced me to the congregation of about sixty-five parishioners. He explained a little about Madonna House and invited me to say a few words. Then he and others presented me with gifts for our Magadan community. A communal meal followed, with more questions and discussion, and more gifts. He would have readily given us a real icon for our chapel, but lacking the necessary documentation, we feared there might be problems getting it across the border.

I left Karsava, my heart singing with indescribable joy. My body was a wreck, but I felt as if my spirit had been renewed in the Lord. I was ready to go home. For the first time since coming to live in Russia, I was eager to return to Magadan. I was eager to see my sisters and Fr. Michael, to share with them this new spiritual friendship, and to continue with them our adventures in the Lord.

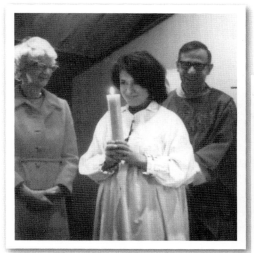

Connie Young, Miriam, Fr. Brière

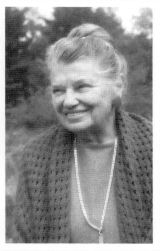

Catherine Doherty

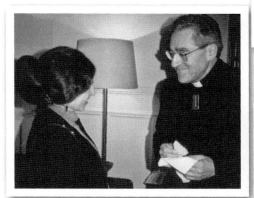

Miriam and Cardinal Lustiger

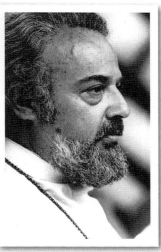

Fr. Alexander Men

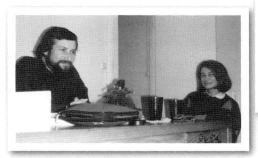

Raia and Volodya at Madonna House Paris

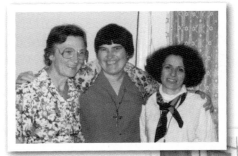

Marie, Alma, and Miriam

Our apartment building
in Magadan

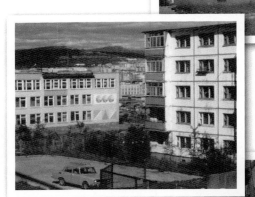

View from our
kitchen window

Miriam packing Russian
Poustinia for shipping

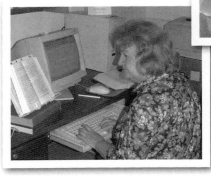

Alvina working on
Russian translations

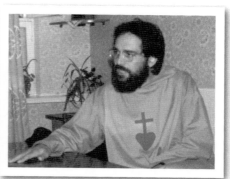

Fr. Michael Shields

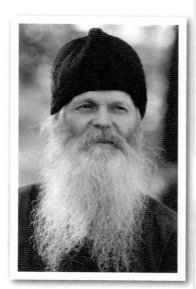

Fr. Viktor Mamontov

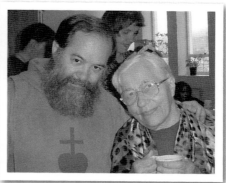

Fr. David and Bronislava

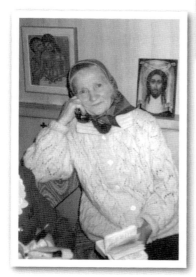

Veronika

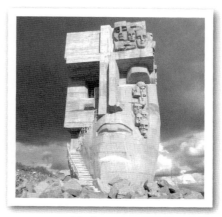

Mask of Sorrow

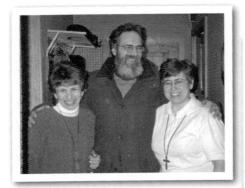

Miriam, Fr. Michael and Sushi

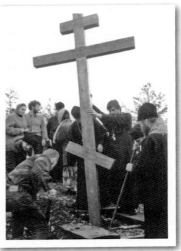

Erecting the cross at Kadikhchan

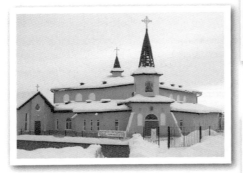

Catholic Church of the Nativity of Christ
in Magadan

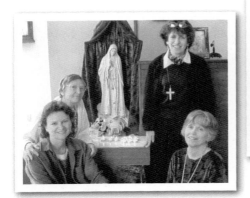

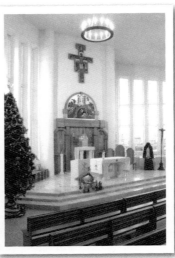

Interior of church

Marie, Katia, Miriam and Liza, 2005

In the Shadow of the Camps

Prayer in atonement for the destruction of Russia's churches and for the suffering perpetrated during the Stalinist years was an integral part of our house mandate. The longer we lived in the Kolyma region, the more we realized how deeply its history was embedded in the lives of our Magadan friends.

One day Alma and I joined our friend Polina for a long walk beyond the Magadanka River. As we chatted, I asked Polina if she felt a personal relationship with the region's past.

"I will tell you about my family," she began. At the time of the Russian Revolution, her great-grandfather had been a prosperous peasant in Ukraine. Twice, everything had been taken from him, and finally, during the brutal collectivization of 1930, the entire family was turned out of their home and sent into exile to Archangelsk, in the far north. Her great-grandfather had refused to leave, saying he was too old to begin again and preferred to die on his own land. He moved into the dog kennels, and Polina believes he starved to death in the subsequent famine. Other family members died in exile. Her grandfather ended up in a labour camp in Kolyma.

"In answer to your question, Miriam" she concluded, "*every* aspect of my life and my family's life is related to the history of Magadan." She paused, and then added quietly, "Russia was a Christian country. I will never understand how she could destroy her own churches, burn her own icons, and kill her own people."

Zina, another of our friends, had grown up next to a women's camp north of Magadan. Her father, a physician, died before she was born. He had been brought to Kolyma to work in the uranium mines where, unprotected from the radioactive dust, prisoners rarely lasted more than six months. Since there was a shortage of doctors, however, he was allowed to exercise his profession and even to be joined by his wife. But his health had already been undermined. Several months before Zina's birth, he was taken away and never heard from again.

Her mother's second husband was a free, salaried worker at the camp. As a child, Zina would overhear him telling her mother about the death of this or that imprisoned writer, musician, or scientist.

The camp was closed after Stalin died, but she and her sister would sometimes wander among the deserted buildings, where they saw the punishment cells, blood stains, and other signs of human suffering.

Many years later, reading Vassula Ryden's prophecies about Russia,* Zina came to understand that her homeland was not under a curse, but was "the beloved daughter of God." She realized that the deepest desire of her heart and the meaning of her life consisted in helping Russia to return to Christ.

The history of Magadan was inseparable from that of the camps. The gold resources of Kolyma had been desperately needed to finance Stalin's massive industrialization projects, and the labour required for its extraction was provided by hundreds of thousands of prisoners, transported by train across the Russian continent to Vladivostok and from there by steamship to Magadan. The latter became the administrative center for a network of labour camps and supporting settlements covering a region roughly the size of France.

Political prisoners came to include ingrained Bolsheviks, Socialists, and Trotskyites; anyone Stalin suspected to be a rival or who could possibly be construed as a rival; anyone who had seen too much; anyone who had the courage or the folly to question any aspect of Soviet policy. Also in danger was anyone even suspected of dissent or of having a connection with a dissenter. Relations of detainees were similarly liable to arrest. There were quotas to be filled, and anyone could be accused of anything. The majority of those sentenced to hard labour under the infamous Statute 58 were simply innocent people caught up in the maelstrom of their terrible times.

The Kolyma camps were particularly dreaded because of the extreme climatic conditions. Only when the temperature dropped below minus fifty degrees Celsius did outdoor work cease, but thermometers were read by camp officials and not subject to verification. Prisoners died by the thousands from exposure, hunger, disease, and exhaustion.

Confessors of the faith

At the end of World War II, the labour camp populations were swelled by returning prisoners-of-war, arrested as traitors simply for having survived capture. Added to their numbers were many Balts

---

* See Vassula Ryden, *True Life in God.*

and Ukrainians, accused of resisting their countries' absorption into the Soviet Union. Among the Lithuanians sentenced at that time to hard labour in Magadan were twenty-five-year-old Veronika and eighteen-year-old Bronislava. Peasant girls accustomed to heavy farm labour, their youthful constitutions helped them survive the gruelling physical conditions, and their staunch Catholic faith was a support in retaining personal integrity.

Among our parish treasures was a rosary Bronislava had made in the camps from bits of dried bread. She and other Catholic prisoners would put aside some of their meagre ration to be rolled into tiny balls and strung on threads unravelled from their clothing. Bronislava later made a replica for Madonna House.

A young woman journalist once interviewed some of the camp survivors from the parish and decided to test Bronislava on the subject of forgiveness. Bronislava had been talking about a particularly sadistic interrogator, saying she would like to meet him again, "just to look him in the eye—not with anger, not to spit at him, but just to know how a person could relate to a human being he had tortured."

"Suppose this interrogator suddenly appeared next to you at Mass," the journalist said, "would you be able to give him your hand at the sign of peace?"

Bronislava was quiet for a few seconds. Then she said softly, but with conviction, "Yes, I would. Yes, of course, I would give him my hand. As I told you, I would like to see him just to know how he could live among people he himself had tortured, but I don't hold anything against him in my heart. I've never cursed anyone. How can I explain this to you? Fr. Michael just said in his homily that we have to forgive those who wrong us. Of course, it's difficult, but what else can we do? God asks it of us. If we hate, if we curse, what good can come of it? We are believers. Maybe someone without faith can hate and swear, but we have faith. It was faith that saved us. If we live in faith, then we have to forgive. This is the way I was raised."

Even after completing their sentences, political prisoners were not allowed to return to their homes. Deprived of civil rights for a given number of years, they were obliged to remain in the Magadan area and report regularly to the authorities. Both Bronislava and

Veronika had married men they met in the camps, non-Lithuanians, and had raised their children in Magadan.

Former prisoners continued to be viewed with suspicion even after the fall of communism. More than once we heard our own parishioners say, "If they were arrested, they must have done something wrong!" Soviet indoctrination had done its work.

Above all else, Bronislava and Veronika strove to pass on to their children the Catholic faith that was their heritage. Veronika herself baptized her son and daughter. Bronislava enlisted the services of a priest newly liberated from the camps. Conscious of their vulnerability as convicted "enemies of the people," both mothers were careful about what they told their children. Veronika said to her daughter, Nelly, "Always remember that you are a baptized Roman Catholic. You must never have any other faith. But never mention it to anyone. I was in the camps, and they can arrest us again."

In 1992 Bronislava heard on the radio that a Catholic Mass was being celebrated each week at the House of Culture. She thought the announcer was probably mistaken, but just to be sure, she decided to go and see for herself. Realizing it was truly a Roman Catholic Mass, she wept for joy.

Both Fr. Austin and Fr. Michael considered these women to be the spiritual pillars of our young parish community. The Parish of the Nativity of Christ was built on the faith of Veronika, Bronislava, and others like them—on their prayers, their faithfulness, and their suffering. They were our treasures.

Our relationship with Aquilina was never as intimate or sustained as our friendships with Veronika and Bronislava, but each encounter left an indelible impression. Tiny, stooped, her wizened face and blue eyes framed by a white, flowered Russian shawl, she appeared at our apartment one evening for the weekly rosary gathering. We had no idea who she was or how she had found us. While she mumbled the prayers, she didn't seem familiar with the Catholic rosary. A little later, two Baptist acquaintances arrived and told us they had arranged to meet Aquilina here.

After the rosary, as we all sat around the table sipping tea and munching cookies, Aquilina began telling her story. Born in Ukraine, she belonged to the True Orthodox Church, also called the Church of the Catacombs, which had gone underground in 1927 in protest of Metropolitan Sergei's decision to include in the Orthodox litany a petition for the Soviet government. The most radical branches of this Church refused any form of cooperation with the Communist regime, which they held to be the Antichrist. Aquilina's family would not register with the government, enrol in schools, join the collective farms, or even sign official documents. During the famine of 1933, deliberately induced by the Soviet government to subdue the peasants and which resulted in over seven million deaths in Ukraine and other parts of the USSR, Aquilina's parents and several siblings perished of starvation. In 1947 eighteen-year-old Aquilina was arrested with her sister and given a ten-year sentence.

She told us story after story of her miraculous survival. As punishment for refusing to work on Easter, she was stripped naked and made to stand outside for five days in sub-freezing temperatures. Overcome by the cold, she thought she was going to die and began to pray to the Trinity, Our Lady, all the saints, and even the stars and the earth. Transfixed, we listened as she repeated for us this litany as fervently and emotionally as she must have prayed it in the camp. Then she described how a great blanket of warmth had enveloped her so that she ceased to feel the cold and even began to perspire.

Another time, in weather of minus sixty degrees Celsius, her whole group had been locked in their barracks because of insubordination. Forbidden to light the stove, they were given one cup of hot tea and three hundred grams of bread a day and were taunted by the guards. Miraculously, they survived. An inspection commission, all bundled up in fur coats and hats, arrived from Moscow to see them. When one of the officers tried to warm his hands at the stove, he was shocked to find it cold. As he left the barracks, the prisoners heard him muttering, "Maybe there is a God, after all!"

Every couple of years, Aquilina would appear at our door. We would gather around her, and she would again tell us her story, the details of which never varied. Each time it happened, we felt as if we had been visited by one of God's holy ones.

Wiping the feet of Christ

I was haunted by the camps. To be raised as a Jew, even in America, was to have the memory of the Holocaust seared into my consciousness. During my time in France, I came to know Jews and

Jewish Christians who had been in concentration camps, and all that I learned and heard went deep into my heart. Something more had to happen, though. I could not hear these stories without searching for their relationship to my own life, which had been so protected and privileged.

In Magadan, we were called to walk reverently before experiences we could not pretend to understand. We listened, trying not to ask questions for the purpose of satisfying our own curiosity. Our goal was not to "look at," but to "stand with." We learned by loving.

Bronislava, Veronika, and others like them were our friends and our mentors. We were humbled by the privilege of being able to serve them, and their trust and friendship were our greatest treasures. In them, we felt as if we were wiping the feet of Christ.

Alma said, "They have suffered so much that we can never do enough for them." I would watch her slide into the seat beside Bronislava at daily Mass, and next to Veronika on Sundays. She never missed an opportunity to help them.

Pilgrimage to the camps

In June 1996 Alma was invited by Tanya Kononova to accompany her and her sons on a two-month journey to Moscow and Ukraine. Shortly after their departure, Marie and I participated in a mini-pilgrimage to the new monument, "Mask of Sorrow," on the outskirts of the city. It had recently been dedicated to the memory of those who had died in the camps. Ten parishioners and Fr. Michael squeezed into a minibus that deposited us halfway up the hill crowned by the giant sculpture. The monument was reached by climbing a long outdoor staircase flanked by stone plaques set in the earth and engraved with the names of Kolyma labour camps.

Commissioned from a Russian émigré sculptor, the granite monument was in the form of a mask-face fifty metres high, divided down the center by a cross. Tumbling down like tears from the left eye were smaller faces. Along the right side of the face, a curved staircase led to an inner room that had been made to resemble an isolation cell. Above it, in place of the right eye, was a window-like opening, cut into the stone from front to back, in which hung a bell from one of the camps.

The back of the monument was hollowed out. Into it was set a huge stone cross on which was crucified a writhing, muscular, iron figure. I didn't like it. The figure was not Christ offering his death so that all men might live through him, but a human being rebelling against his fate. The one symbol capable of expressing and bestowing meaning on an otherwise inadmissible suffering had been appropriated and misconstrued.

Our little group gathered in front of the monument to pray the rosary for those who had died in the camps. Behind us was Nagayevo Bay. Bronislava had attended the official dedication of the memorial the week before. She told us now that as she had watched the long line of people filing up the hill to the monument, she had had a sudden flashback to her own arrival in Magadan, when she and the other prisoners had been marched from the port to a transit camp at the foot of this same hill.

That she would speak of this was significant. Notwithstanding the controversies surrounding the monument's political, aesthetic, and spiritual qualities, its very existence helped to legitimate the suffering of Bronislava and other camp survivors, finally enabling them to speak openly of the past. At a library gathering with the victims of the repression, one of them told the organizers, "Thank you for giving us the right to be human beings again."

On another day Marie, Fr. Michael, and I took a bus to an abandoned village on Gertner Bay, on the other side of the city. We walked for about forty-five minutes along a path overlooking the sea to a site that had most recently been a children's summer camp, but which had previously been used by the army. Fr. Michael thought it might originally have served as a prison. Some of the barracks, in various states of disrepair, were still extant, with bars on the windows and thick locks on the doors.

We climbed one of the watchtowers. Fr. Michael dragged a heavy table from the enclosure to the tower deck, and on this makeshift altar, he celebrated Mass for the victims of the Kolyma camps. Whether or not this particular camp had been part of the gulag, it became for us a place where we could lift up all the pain of Russia, Kolyma, and our own lives as well, uniting that pain to Christ's sacrifice and offering our lives in reparation for what had happened in this land.

During these weeks we were inwardly preparing for a pilgrimage with Bishop Rastislav and members of his clergy to the sites of some of the former labour camps. Fr. Tikhon, the superior of the Orthodox monastery near Magadan, had invited Fr. Michael to come along. When Lyuba realized how much Marie and I also wanted to come, she mentioned it to Fr. Tikhon, who, in turn, spoke to the bishop. A week later Lyuba phoned to say that Vladika had given permission for us to join the group. We could hardly believe our good fortune! We were told that the trip would be rugged and that we should bring along enough food for three days.

July seventeenth, the anniversary of the assassination of Tsar Nicholas II and his family, had been declared a day of remembrance throughout Russia. We attended the Divine Liturgy at the Orthodox church, followed by a *panikhida,* a prayer service for the dead, offered for those who had died during the Stalinist repression and especially in the camps of Kolyma. Bishop Rastislav spoke eloquently and requested prayers for the forthcoming pilgrimage.

Two days later, with Fr. Michael carrying our heavy bottles of water and juice, as well as a big thermos of tea, we left our house at 6:30 A.M. in a light drizzle. When we got to the Orthodox church, the pastor invited us to wait in the parish kitchen, where we were soon joined by two young women. Marie and I were relieved to discover we would not be the only females on the pilgrimage.

When the bus provided by the city arrived, we quickly piled in and started off, collecting more priests and seminarians along the way. By the time everyone was aboard, all eighteen seats were occupied.

Just two hours out of Magadan, there was a loud crash as a bag at the back of the bus fell heavily to the floor and lay there with steam gushing forth. The bag was ours, and hot tea from the broken thermos was soaking the backpack and its contents. Marie and I pitched the thermos and mopped up the mess, not daring to look at Fr. Michael, several rows behind us. So much for wanting to be inconspicuous!

We began to sort out our travelling companions. There were five bearded priests in soutanes, all younger than Fr. Michael, who was forty-seven. Two had been ordained by the previous bishop. The others, friends of Vladika and of each other, had come from Moscow.

Like Vladika, they were university graduates. Alexei, a young married deacon, was keeping things organized with quiet authority

The two young women were members of the choir. A third woman, the choir director, joined us later that day in Yagodnoye. The girls were wearing dark skirts, long-sleeved blouses, and head-scarves, and we were glad we had decided to dress as discreetly as possible ourselves.

Completing the group were four seminarians from Holy Trinity Monastery near Moscow, founded in the fourteenth century by St. Sergei of Radonezh; a novice from Fr. Tikhon's monastery, a TV cameraman who had worked for Fr. Austin and was now working with the Orthodox parish, and his young helper. Travelling separately and scheduled to join us the next morning were Bishop Rastislav with two more priests.

Gradually, we began to get acquainted. Two of the seminarians insisted that Marie and I exchange places with them, as we had selected a particularly bumpy spot above one of the rear wheels. Fr. Michael, in the back seat next to the ever-smiling Fr. Vasily, quickly became the object of lively questioning about everything from the Latin liturgy to Madonna House. We prayed for him as he stumbled along in broken Russian—his linguistic limitations had no bearing on the significance of this sharing. We watched him pull from his backpack a breviary, rosary booklet, Bible, and other prayer books. All were eagerly passed around and examined by his companions. When we heard him haltingly pronouncing prayers in Church Slavonic, we were moved at his humble simplicity.

Marie and I were treated with exquisite courtesy. As laywomen, we were not expected to answer the kinds of theological and ecumenical questions Fr. Michael was being bombarded with. Most of the questions asked of us had to do with America, but as neither of us had lived there for years, our answers could not have been very enlightening. Once, when a young seminarian with thick slanting brows and a burning curiosity began asking our opinion of projected religious legislation, Deacon Alexei came to our rescue and quietly drew him away.

It was clear to Marie, Fr. Michael, and me that what really mattered was not our stumbling responses to questions, but the shared experiences of these four days, the shattering of stereotypes, and coming to know each other as persons. That Vladika had invited us was a public expression of his regard for the Catholic Church. Most important of all was the intense, shared prayer of these days. The barriers were not all breached, but as Fr. Michael observed afterwards, "At least they know we are believers."

We had been warned that there would be no food or toilet facilities until we reached Yagodnoye early that evening. Indeed, all we saw along the way were abandoned villages. These settlements had originally been built to serve the camps or to supply trucks along the thousand-kilometre Kolyma highway. The entire region had been supported by the central government in return for its gold, and now that this support was no longer forthcoming, the area was dying. Most of the villages had been officially closed. The abandoned buildings were in various stages of dismantlement, the wood torn away to be used for fuel or building material. It was a depressing sight, but our sadness was mixed with a sense that this process was inevitable—the life of the region had been built on a foundation that was intrinsically evil.

Yagodnoye had once been a pleasant, medium-sized town, but during our first winter in Magadan, an accident at the nearby power plant had left the town without heat in minus thirty degree cold. Children and old people were evacuated. Frozen pipes having caused widespread damage, many families moved away. Everywhere we saw empty buildings.

As the restaurant where we were to have supper was not yet ready to serve us, it was decided to celebrate a memorial service, or *panikhida*, at the tomb of a bishop who had died in the camps. Marie and I missed it! With the other women on the bus, we had gone with a local resident to use the bathroom in her apartment several streets away, and by the time we returned, the bus had already left for the cemetery. We waited in the little church with one of the priests, who had fallen into a pool at the foot of a waterfall where we stopped for lunch, and was still wet. Since it was now raining steadily, the others had convinced him to stay where it was warm.

The Yagodnoye church was actually a small house in the first stages of remodelling. Wires hung from the ceiling and projected out from the walls, and paper reproductions of icons were tacked to the unfinished plywood iconostasis. Even so, there was everything necessary for the liturgy, and vespers was celebrated as soon as the bus returned. We went back to the restaurant, and after a quick supper, we were taken to a student dormitory—now empty, since it was summer—where we were to spend the night. We managed to convince the lady who got us all settled that it was better for the women to have a different bathroom from the priests and seminarians. By the time we turned out the light, it was well past midnight.

The next day was Saturday. There had been some confusion about what time the liturgy would begin, and since Marie and I were never too sure in any case about what was to happen at any given time, we were up long before the bus arrived to take us to the church.

The service included matins, the small hours, the blessing of holy water, and the Divine Liturgy. Deacon Alexei said we should feel free to go out and rest whenever we felt the need. Oh, no, I protested, that wouldn't be necessary. Shortly afterwards, I almost fainted from the combined effects of incense, lack of sleep, and an empty stomach. He sent us both to the bus with instructions to have something to eat since we weren't receiving communion.

Somewhat to our embarrassment, we were still in the bus when Vladika's jeep pulled up beside us. He had been detained in Magadan by a funeral and had arrived in Yagodnoye during the night. Some of the priests came out to greet him, and we were moved at the warmth with which he welcomed Fr. Michael.

The clergy of the Magadan eparchy* crowded into the unfinished chapel for the Divine Liturgy, along with a dozen or so local people. By the time we went for lunch at the restaurant where we had eaten the night before, it was at least twelve-thirty. Deacon Alexei had checked beforehand to see if we ate meat. Vladika invited Fr. Michael to accompany him in his jeep on the return trip, taking the long route home through more camp sites. It was a beautiful gesture, even though it didn't work out in the end because the heavy rains had washed out the road they were to take.

After lunch, as we waited in the bus to leave for the Serpentinka death camp, a grizzled old man climbed aboard, leaning heavily on his cane. His long, brown cape and soutane were dirty. He looked like a *yourodivyi*, a "fool for Christ." It was the legendary Fr. Nikolai,

---

* *Eparchy* – the Orthodox equivalent to a diocese.

who had served in the same camp as his bishop, for whom the *pan-ikhida* had been sung the previous evening. After his own release, Fr. Nikolai had brought the bishop's bones to Yagodnoye for reburial. Both of the chapels he had built there were confiscated by the government. When Fr. Nikolai's house burned to the ground, Bishop Rastislav invited him to Magadan, but Fr. Nikolai chose instead to move to an old age home nearby in order to spend his last days in the area where he had lived for so long,.

He had come now to greet the priests, who gathered around him with great respect. Marie and I had long wanted to meet this man about whom we had heard so much. Although we remained in the rear of the bus, we were still moved.

The drive to Serpentinka, over switchback mountain roads, took an hour. The land felt deserted. Not a trace remained of the camp, the rumoured existence of which had aroused such terror in the Kolyma prisoners. Those sentenced to death had been brought here for execution. Jammed tightly together in a barrack to await nightfall, they were then called out in groups of five. Revved-up tractor motors muffled the revolver shots. A man who somehow escaped execution wrote that seventy people would be killed in a single night. Someone else estimated that thirty thousand were shot in the course of a year.

After only two years the camp was closed, razed to the ground, and its entire staff executed. The location was rediscovered years later when miners, washing gold in the stream that had once run through the camp, came upon human bones.

Above the quiet valley, a simple stone memorial stood on a grassy incline. Behind it was a cross, erected by a man whose father had been shot at Serpentinka. Next to the father's name and dates of birth and death was engraved the name and Moscow telephone number of his son, a tacit invitation for anyone with information about the father to contact the family.

Vladika was already waiting by the memorial when our bus arrived. Quickly, we gathered around him, scrambling up the incline. Wearing his black, wide-sleeved soutane, stole, and brimless blue velvet cap, he began the service for the dead. It was as if there was nothing in him but prayer, washing like a tide across the horrors of history. The patriarch had asked that *panikhidas* be celebrated in all the former gulag sites of Russia, and during these days of pilgrimage, it was as if this little group of black-robed priests, swinging their censors and led by their red-haired bishop, were redeeming the blasphemed land for God.

As the deceased were commended to the mercy of Christ, a peace seemed to settle over the valley. After the concluding hymn, *Vechnaya pamyat*–"Eternal Memory"–Vladika reminded us that this eternal remembrance of the dead belonged to God, not to us. Human memory, in most cases, embraced only a few generations, but God held each of us in his hand, now and forever. Not one person was lost or abandoned. *Each hair of your head has been counted.* (Mt 10:30)

It came to me that my presence here as a Jewish Christian was no coincidence. God had brought me to this place and to this hour from France, from Combermere, from my American childhood, to pray for the Jewish dead of Kolyma so that they too might be brought out of nameless oblivion into the eternal remembrance of God. I recalled the words of the *Kaddish*, the traditional Jewish prayer for the deceased that includes no mention of death, but is a proclamation of faith in God's greatness: "*Magnified and sanctified be his great name in the world which he has created according to his will...Blessed, praised and glorified, exalted, extolled and honoured, magnified and lauded be the name of the Holy One, blessed be he...*." Standing again so unexpectedly in the stream of Jewish history, I knew that the sufferings of my own people were meant to open my heart to all suffering.

After the *panikhida*, some of the group went down into the valley and walked along the stream. I waited until the others were far ahead. I didn't want to talk to anyone yet. Then I walked down and stood without moving for a long time. I wept.

The sun was shining. The valley was empty, peaceful, silent except for the singing of the stream. There was not a trace of the agony, the fear, the cries, the despair.

> *The souls of the just are in the hands of God,*
> *no torment shall ever touch them.*
> *In the eyes of the universe, they did appear to die,*
> *their agony looked like a disaster,*
> *their leaving us, an annihilation;*
> *but they are at peace...* (Wisdom 3:19)

I went back up the hill. At the foot of the memorial were bouquets of wild flowers and scattered coins. I wanted to leave something too, but the only object I had with me was the cord rosary a Filipino poustinik had given me in Paris and that I usually carried in my pocket. I kissed it and placed it next to the flowers. When I told Marie what I had done, she took from her bag a medal of St. Maximilian Kolbe, the martyr of Auschwitz, and added it to the little pile of offerings. Later she helped Vladika fill a small plastic bag with earth from Serpentinka. I wished that we too could have taken home some earth, but we had no container to put it in.

From Serpentinka we set off for Susuman, where we were to spend the night. It would have been a three-hour trip had there not been engine trouble. The driver fiddled with it, we chugged along for a bit, and then the bus broke down definitively. A truck with chains pulled us off the road, after which there was nothing to do but relax and wait for help. Fortunately, the sun had come out, and by pooling what food was left, we had enough for tea. No one complained. In Russia, such problems were too frequent not to be accepted philosophically.

We strolled along the road and up the mountainside, enjoying the warmth and the scenery. In other places, the country had been disfigured by piles of slag left from strip mining, but here the mountain slopes were covered with fields upon fields of purple fireweed. The brief Kolyma summer was at its height, with a splendid profusion and variety of wild flowers. So idyllic was the setting that it would have been easy to forget what had brought us here.

Marie and I never knew where the replacement bus came from. Leaving our original driver sitting on the step of his broken vehicle, two loaves of bread at his side, we all transferred our luggage to the second bus.

With the summer days stretching later and later as we travelled north, it was still bright daylight when we reached Susuman at 10 P.M. Vladika had arrived earlier in his jeep, and vespers was already under way. In contrast to the little church in Yagodnoye, this one was fully constructed, its walls lined with real icons. A priest was in permanent residence. Marie and I were so warmly welcomed by one of the women that we wondered if we had met her somewhere before, but it was a manifestation of the hospitality lavished upon our whole group. That some of us were Catholics made no difference.

After the liturgy we were escorted across the street to an apartment where an abundant supper had been prepared. It must have been close to 1 A.M. before we got to the hotel. Clean and freshly-painted, it was quite an improvement over the dormitory where we had spent the previous night. This time we stayed with the two choir members in a room that had hot and cold water, a shower, and a toilet. That the latter had to be flushed from a bucket was only a minor inconvenience. Gratefully, we washed off the dirt of the road. There had been so much dust that each time a vehicle passed us, someone had to jump up and close the vent in the roof of the bus—our only source of ventilation. By the time we fell into bed, it was 2 A.M.

Sunday morning began with the Divine Liturgy. The tiny church was filled with parishioners, and Vladika Rastislav gave a moving homily in which he explained the reason for our trip. We were not only praying for the Kolyma dead, he reminded them, but also soliciting their prayers, the powerful prayers of martyrs.

Throughout this trip Marie and I were continually impressed by the spiritual authority of this young bishop. His parents had been atheists, but the religious formation he received from his grandmother became the foundation for his future calling. At Moscow University he earned a degree in literature. When the churches were at last permitted to function freely, he entered Holy Trinity Monastery at Zagorsk, was ordained to the priesthood, taught at the seminary, and despite his youth, became a spiritual father to quite a number of people. Attracting the attention of the patriarch, he was asked in 1993 to become bishop of the Magadan eparchy. Others had already refused the appointment. Fr. Rastislav had no desire to leave his monastery, but each time he broached the subject with his spiritual father, the latter was noncommittal: "Magadan…a place of suffering…cold… the cross…" Fr. Rastislav accepted God's invitation.

His presence was transforming the eparchy. Our own Bishop Werth, during his last visit to Magadan, had met Vladika and some of the priests he had brought from Moscow and had been impressed by this new model of educated, cultured Orthodox clergy.

Nowhere was Vladika's spiritual intensity more tangible than at Kadikhchan, two hours northeast of Susuman. After lunch, climbing onto yet another bus, we drove through barren, forbidding, empty countryside, not far from the border of the neighbouring republic of Yakutia.* The sky was dark and threatening, matching the desolation of the landscape. We couldn't find the place where we were to meet Vladika and drove up one road, then down another. Just as we were about to head back to the ramshackle settlement to ask for directions, we spotted a huge, wooden Orthodox cross lying against a slope and the bishop's jeep parked nearby.

Never will I forget that spot. Never will I forget the power of God's presence through the liturgical prayer. It pierced my soul. It seemed to pierce the very universe.

The labour camp had stood in the valley; we could see in the distance the mining settlement that had succeeded it. We were standing at the edge of a river, next to a concrete bunker-type structure jutting out from the hill. Its entrance seemed to be a low tunnel leading into the hill itself. Even now, in mid-July, the ground inside was covered with ice. The structure had served as a *kartzer*, or punishment cell. Men were sentenced to spend one or more days in this cramped space without food, water, or heat. In icy winter temperatures, they froze to death within hours.

I was overwhelmed by a sense of evil, the magnitude of which I had never experienced. Cold, clutching, all-encompassing evil. I wanted to cry out against it, but it was like being in a nightmare where the scream freezes in one's throat. It wasn't just the weather, the cold wind, or the rain that began to fall. It was the kind of evil against which man, if he relies on his own resources, is powerless.

At the edge of the river, Vladika celebrated a short prayer service for the blessing of water. Three times he dipped a small cross into the stream. Then he filled two plastic cups with water. Someone passed one of the cups to Fr. Michael to hold as we all scrambled up the incline to where the giant cross lay. We clustered around Vladika as he began the next set of prayers, blessing the cross with the holy water. At a gesture from the bishop, the priests hoisted the cross onto their shoulders and all but ran with it up the hill. The rest of us followed.

* The Russian Federation consists of 21 republics, 48 provinces, 7 territories, one autonomous region, and 7 autonomous districts. The republic of Yakutia (Sakha) is the largest in geographical territory.

Near the top, where a hole had been prepared, the cross was inserted and provisionally secured.

The ensuing *panikhida* was like a burial rite for those whose bones lay in the bowels of the hill or scattered across the valley. Planted above them now was the sign of Christ's victory. Our eyes riveted to the cross, we sang the now-familiar chants in Church Slavonic.

Suddenly I understood. The abandonment of man to the powers of destruction that loomed in these skies had been broken forever on Golgotha. The men left to die in the frozen darkness of these hillside cells had not been alone. The horror of having one's existence blotted out forever, ground into the blackness, could not be the ultimate conclusion. Whether or not they had been conscious of him, Christ had been at their side in the terror of those final hours.

I understood now why we had to let ourselves be broken and humiliated. It was because he had come to them not as a victor, but as the crucified one, the suffering one, the humiliated one. There was no place on earth or under the earth where his mercy and love could not penetrate.

The rain was falling harder and harder. Lightning flashed, but no one moved until the final prayer had been intoned. Vladika, followed first by the priests and then by the rest of us, turned a shovelful of dirt and stones into the hole where the cross had been inserted. When it was secure, we came forward, one by one, to kiss the cross. I touched to it my own Madonna House cross.

The sense of oppression was gone. The rain became lighter and then stopped altogether. The sun broke through the clouds, bathing the hill in sunshine.

We went back to the bus, and as the driver pulled onto the main road, we kept turning for a last glimpse of the Cross of Christ, silhouetted against the sky.

Back in Susuman, we were fed again and sent to rest at the hotel for a few hours until the arrival of the replacement bus, sent by the Yagodnoye administration. The first bus had seemed modest, but it was luxurious compared to the little school bus into which we crowded for the return trip to Magadan.

Once again it was raining. During the four-hour drive to Yagodnoye, both fan belts broke. We waited an hour in Yagodnoye for replacements to be found and fitted, but they too came loose on the way back to Magadan. When the windshield wipers developed problems, the driver of our first bus, who was riding with us, worked them manually throughout the night.

It was a long trip home, eighteen hours over uneven roads, with rain now dribbling down *inside* the bus windows. Not much conversation—everyone was too tired. We mostly dozed. Our Susuman hosts had sent us off with bags of food and drink, which we passed around at appropriate intervals. At various points we stopped to relieve ourselves under the bushes in the rain.

Around noon the next day the rain finally ceased, and we pulled up at a scenic spot to stretch our legs. Marie and one of the priests found a family of groundhogs living in the ruins of an abandoned hut. Fr. Vasily presented us with an armful of wildflowers he had gathered.

The bus arrived in Magadan at about 3 P.M. Some of the priests had been dropped off along the way at the villages where they lived. Fr. Michael, Marie, and I got off near the parish chapel and walked to our apartment. In our Madonna House chapel, Fr. Michael celebrated Mass for the first time in four days, and for the first time in four days we were able to receive communion.

The spiritual impact of Kadikhchan, of Vladika Rastislav raising the cross over a valley reeking of evil and claiming Christ's victory, had been so powerful that it was several days before I could think of it without tears coming to my eyes. Nor could I speak of it without my voice breaking. It was one of the strongest experiences I had ever had. I prayed that it would change my life.

Going to the Poor, Being Poor

By 1996 we were making a conscious effort to reach out to the poor. Marie was convinced that we needed to move in this direction. It also kept the apostolate from becoming too narrowly identified with one group, the core of active parishioners who continually sought us out.

We tried to emulate our Russian friends, who never refused food or help to anyone who asked. When our efforts stretched us almost to the breaking point, we learned what it meant to live by grace. We were being challenged to live the Gospel without compromise, and it was a precious opportunity.

It was easy for me to relate to our more educated friends, who were delighted by my interest in Russian poetry and culture. Marie encouraged this, but at the same time, she felt it was important for me to keep reaching out to those I found more difficult to accept. God could not have tailored for me a more appropriate school of purification.

When I told Fr. Michael I felt no attraction to the poor, he said, "You are being called to do what you don't do well. The only way to learn to love is to love badly."

One Sunday morning our little, wrinkled, henna-haired neighbour, Miroslava, arrived while we were getting dressed for Mass. When we didn't stop to give her our undivided attention, she felt unwelcome and left in a huff.

"We have to be careful with the little ones," Marie said. "They are precious."

"Even when they are eating us up?" I protested.

"We have a vow of poverty. On a material level, we can't live as poorly as the people here, so we have to become poor this way."

Once again, her words cut through the controls, the brakes, the conditions I desperately sought to impose upon our life. Once again, I touched the bitter knowledge of my inner refusal and instinctive negativity. Miroslava's demands might have been unreasonable, but reasonableness, in this case, didn't seem to be a criterion. We were being called to love without counting the cost, accepting whatever was asked of us and whomever God sent.

The vision to which we were being called was terrifying, but when I fell on my knees before the Blessed Sacrament, when I left the isolation of my cerebral, egocentric self and opened my heart to Jesus, the resistance fell away. I had already chosen to follow him, and there was nothing to go back to. I no longer had any life but Christ.

Pure physical fatigue was where I was most vulnerable. Exhaustion seemed to be our constant companion, but Marie and Alma had more natural energy than I did. We were going to bed late each night; I'd been sleeping badly and waking up early. I feared and hated the loss of perspective and emotional control that accompanied fatigue. I resented the absence of boundaries in our life that exacted such a price.

Normally, I would have talked it out with Marie, but something in me said, "Don't do that just now. God is calling you to total surrender. Give it all to Our Lady, and trust her to give you what you need."

It seemed pretty radical, but I made an act of faith. When the following day, Sunday, was also non-stop, Marie declared a sleep-in and free morning for Monday. I only slept until eight-thirty but awoke refreshed, prayed leisurely, and felt as if Our Lady had answered my prayer. Although I had initiated nothing, she was taking care of me. Lightness and joy filled my heart. It was an important lesson, and I wrote in my journal:

> God brought me to the edge, rescued me, and is calling me to live on this edge, dependent on him alone. The Spirit is leading. *Lord, help me not to resist you.*

Living the Gospel without compromise

From our friends came forceful examples of the Gospel living to which we aspired. They were not afraid of its absoluteness and did not adjust its standard to their ability to respond. They took leaps of faith that left us breathless.

There was Nina, who taught at the choir school behind our apartment and who by now had become a close friend. She had told me about her problems with a former student, Daniela. Somewhat masculine in manner and dress, and obviously disturbed, Daniela had started coming to Saturday evening Mass. According to Nina, Daniela had been "pursuing her" for years, trying to insinuate herself into Nina's family circle. And now she had followed her to church!

Nina was almost desperate. Her son Toli was in prison, awaiting trial. The church was her refuge, and now it was being invaded. I felt sorry for her, but what could I say? That the Gospel calls us to love our enemies?

On Saturday evenings, Nina and I led the singing. One night, toward the end of the homily, she leaned over and whispered to me, "Watch!" I had no idea what she was going to do. As people stood to offer their prayer intentions, Nina slid out from behind the electronic organ, moved quietly to where Daniela was sitting several rows in front of us, tapped her on the shoulder, and beckoned her back to sing with us in the choir. I couldn't believe what I was seeing. The whole-heartedness of that act, fraught with personal consequences— an act done in pure obedience to the Gospel I hadn't had the courage to preach—overwhelmed and convicted me.

Some time later, Fr. Michael told Polina, the regular parish organist, that he wanted to start paying her for her services. Although she hadn't received her teaching salary for several months and was in acute need of money, she refused. Music was the gift God had given her, and she wanted to offer it back gratuitously. Only in Russia does this make sense, I thought.

The desire to love with this kind of totality was growing in my heart. So much of my spiritual approach was governed by the North American preoccupation with psychology and focused not on Christ, but on myself. In contrast to Nina and Polina, who could take such spiritual leaps, I felt mired in my emotional patterns, stuck in the same, stale efforts to cope with interpersonal relationships.

Fr. Michael suggested that during Lent, I should try talking to the Lord on the cross. He began showing me "how to live on the cross," as he put it. As a first step, he suggested I try to accept silently what I perceived as personal injustices, try to "taste the cross a little," and to "choose a way of suffering." Each time I felt humiliated or attacked, I should endeavour to stand defenceless. Each time a conflict or disagreement arose, I was to ask forgiveness of the other person.

I was shocked. It was like being asked to stand still in a bull ring, a matador without his cape. Fr. Michael pointed out that defencelessness didn't mean being deserted. God was present, and I needed to pray for faith. "We are called to live in crucified love," he said, "where we have nothing to defend, where we have given up everything, and are nailed helpless. This is our goal."

My only other choice, he added, was to go back to living in my head. I couldn't make myself feel love, but I could let myself feel pain. The two were extremely close. Pain opened the heart.

I wrote to my spiritual director at Madonna House:

> How can one choose to suffer? It goes against everything natural and healthy in a human being. It goes against my humanistic formation, against my former understanding of faith. And the worst of it is that this proposition, which has always shocked and revolted me, against which I have always rebelled, and which seemed to have no place at all in a psychologically healthy world, now looms before me as an invitation, almost a call.
>
> I cannot make a blanket choice. I can't say to God, "Yes, I choose the way of suffering." Nor can I ask him for it. But I have a hunch that one doesn't choose "a way"; one chooses *him*. All I can do is to stand before Christ on the crucifix and say, *I want to be with you. Help me not to be afraid.*

A few entries from my poustinia journal:[*]

June 18, 1996

God is showing me how to live by his grace. This is a new country of the spirit. If he wants this, he'll give me what I need. There is likely to be a price, but I am being taught not to count the cost. This is a time to think big, to keep the vision high.

Acceptance of a challenge does not imply or depend on the ability to live it out. What freedom this is! How is it possible that I've never understood it before?

I am learning to live in the struggle, to feel its pain. In other words, to let life be itself. Isn't this what I've always longed for? God has truly pulled me in over my depth, and

---

[*] Subsequent dated entries are taken from my poustinia journal.

I feel like Peter walking on the water. If I look away from Jesus—game over.

With Alma away in Ukraine for two months and only two of us left, living the impossible has become even more insane. Yesterday at midnight, Marie insisted that we balance our accounts. All I could think was, I hope God appreciates the effort, because at this hour, the figures are never going to add up!

All day yesterday we were besieged by the poor, our "little ones." Will I ever see in them the face of God, as Catherine did, as Marie and Alma and Fr. Michael do? Perhaps it isn't a question of loving "them," but of trying to love Lyubov, Nikola, Kostya.....

July 1, 1996

I stayed home from the White Nights Festival, planning to go to bed early, but Piotr arrived at 10:15 P.M., badly needing to talk, and it was one before I got to bed. Yesterday, Sunday, Marie and I worked on the evening meal all day except for Mass and an hour's rest in the afternoon, since we'd invited Fr. Michael, his two guests from Alaska, and Alvina. Predictably, Lyubov showed up just as we started and joined us. Then, after we'd eaten everything on the table, Matushka Fiokla and Nikola arrived. Marie cooked a second supper for them, and Lyubov devoured it too.

Last week I made a big pot of soup each morning, thinking it would last a few days. Each evening, after we had fed everyone who stopped by, there was barely enough left for supper. "Do you think God wants us to be a restaurant?" Marie wondered plaintively.

How many times this week have I thought, "I can't do this!" But no sooner do the words form themselves than others follow: "Save me, Lord; I'm drowning!" and "Be merciful to me, a sinner." Only by grace can we make it through this summer.

The need to protect myself seems less. The defence mechanisms are still in place, but my faith is stronger, and the panic dissolves more quickly. If I fall apart, I fall apart. That's God's business.

As Marie said, the poverty to which we are called in Magadan is the inability to control our lives. Only if we let go completely can we survive here. I'm not there yet, but I want to be.

July 23, 1996

I am still reeling from the impact of our pilgrimage to Kolyma. Marie and I were both sick for a couple days after we returned. Marie thinks it was either food poisoning or something in the water. In my opinion, the very intensity of the experience was enough to knock us off our feet.

After Kolyma, so much of what I've been struggling with no longer matters –pride, recognition, achievement. It isn't easy to let them go, but their insignificance is clear.

God is saying, "Stand straight in the truth and keep looking at me. Don't get distracted. I am leading you."

Catching a thief

In August Fr. Tom Zoeller arrived from Combermere to spend three weeks with us. He moved gracefully into our non-stop life. One day, when there was no time to prepare meals, we ate a pot of buckwheat under different guises for breakfast, lunch, and supper. Another day, he brought over his dirty laundry in the morning, as Marie had suggested, but took it back in the evening to do himself!

Alma returned from her two-month journey with Tanya and Kirill, but we were unable to meet her plane. The previous afternoon had been like a three-ring-circus. Two young boys, Andrei and Vitya had been working on jigsaw puzzles in the living room while Marie and I were occupied with other guests in the kitchen. At one point Marie went to get money to give someone for medicine. We kept both roubles and dollars in a blue cloth bag under one of the beds, where we could get to it easily, and with all the activity, she had forgotten to hide the sack again.

Not until we were almost ready to go to bed did we discover that the money bag was empty. Of all the people who had been in the house that day, the only ones who could possibly have slipped into the bedroom and taken the cash were Andrei and Vitya.

The next morning Marie awoke with the conviction that we needed to go immediately to confront Andrei and his mother, Natasha, whom he had brought to meet us only the week before. We were out of the house by nine. We knew their apartment building, and since Andrei's mother had told us about their recent fire, we were able to identify their rooms by the charred windows.

The family lived in a communal apartment. A man who turned out to be Andrei's stepfather, Seriozha, let us in and ushered us through a dingy corridor to the kitchen, which they shared with other families. He seated us on two rickety stools and squatted at our feet. Obviously hung-over, he made an effort to focus and to deal with Marie's quietly persistent request to see Andrei's mother. The night before, Seriozha and Natasha had been celebrating four years of living together, and we gathered that she wasn't in much better shape than he was. Marie finally had to tell him why we had come, and that if we couldn't see Natasha, we would be obliged to call the police. Since Natasha seemed to have no intention of coming out of the bedroom, Marie insisted that he bring us in to her.

The room into which Seriozha led us had three beds, a cupboard for clothing, peeling wallpaper, and a bare floor with peeling paint. Clothes were piled here and there and folded over a clothesline that stretched across one corner of the room. In another corner were small paper icons and the Orthodox cross Marie had given Natasha the week before. Religious pictures were pasted on two of the walls.

Andrei's fourteen-year-old sister, Oksana, was still in bed. On the edge of another unmade bed sat Natasha, her head in her hands and a sweater pulled down over her nightdress.

Marie told her about the missing money, which amounted to a considerable sum. Natasha denied that her son would have taken it and insisted that his friend Vitya was the culprit. Seriozha decided to go get Andrei, who was hiding in the bathroom, afraid to come out. Andrei vehemently denied having taken our money, even when Marie confronted him with other, smaller thefts—a flashlight, a penknife, and Alma's keys. He claimed that the bills Natasha had seen the previous evening were his earnings from filling gas tanks with

Vitya. Swearing at his mother, he called her a crazy drunk. Marie had to restrain Natasha from placing a curse on him.

I don't know what would have happened if Vitya's father had not arrived just then. At first, Natasha refused to see him, but Seriozha convinced her and Andrei to come out to the kitchen. We could hear their raised voices. Oksana, who until then hadn't said a word other than, "I *told* him not to bring his friends to see you!" took advantage of the lull to swing out of bed and into her clothes, tossing spreads over all the crumpled bed sheets.

The rest of the family returned. If we correctly understood the explanation, in highly colloquial and not very sober Russian, by the time Vitya's father had discovered the theft, Vitya had already distributed the money among his friends. His father had beaten him mercilessly.

We pointed out to Andrei that as an accessory to the theft, he was just as responsible as Vitya. Natasha, alternating between tears and threats, was threatening to beat Andrei to a pulp. Marie told her not to talk like that. Andrei wasn't a bad boy, but he was weak and easily influenced by bad friends. She told Andrei to come over to her and ask for forgiveness. Finally, he acquiesced.

"I forgive you and God forgives you," said Marie. Then she made him ask forgiveness of his mother.

"I won't forgive him," said Natasha.

"You have to," said Marie.

"I won't."

"You have to forgive him," Marie repeated. We weren't sure if Natasha actually said, "I forgive you," but finally, she hugged the boy.

We prayed the Our Father.

Marie wanted Vitya's father to come see us, but Natasha said it wouldn't happen. She told us she had been baptized in the Orthodox Church and showed us her Bible. Marie opened it at random and read the passage where Jesus casts out an evil spirit that subsequently enters a herd of pigs. Natasha said she had evil spirits herself. On the evidence of the last two hours, Marie was inclined to agree with her.

"You can't afford to pay back the money the boys stole," Marie acknowledged, "so instead, why don't you 'pay it back' by going to confession?"

Natasha was afraid.

"I'll go with you," said Marie.

"You will?"

"Of course I will."

They agreed to meet at our house at ten o'clock Saturday morning, and Marie repeated it on the off-chance that Andrei and Oksana might remember to mention it when the parents sobered up. Our expectations were minimal—so much so that on Saturday, as we went about our weekly cleaning, it was noon before we realized they hadn't shown up.

All this time I had been keeping an eye on the clock. There was no way we could leave gracefully before having hot chocolate and seeing the rest of the communal apartment. In any case, it was already too late to get out to the airport to meet Alma's plane. We got home just before Tanya phoned to say that she, Kirill, and Alma had arrived and would be coming into the city by bus.

Alma was thrilled to be back in Magadan. She described her summer as a time of walking in the footsteps of the crucified Christ. Despite the thousands of kilometres separating us, God had been schooling all three of us in poverty and obedience.

Inching towards the heart

At the beginning of September, after fighting bronchitis for two weeks, I was confined to bed. It was a bad time to be out of commission, for we were in the midst of re-wallpapering the chapel. To make matters worse, my back went out. I found it humiliating not being able to pitch in and even more humiliating not being able to accept the situation gracefully. I was swimming in my poverty.

September 25, 1996

I don't want to be in this position, and no one even has time to sympathize! It is truly a poustinia in the marketplace, and my only real option is obedience and surrender. I am the weakest member of this community, unable to break out of my loneliness, frustration, and self-pity.

Have mercy on me, Lord! I can't move by myself. Give me your grace. Please, please, don't let me refuse it.

September 27, 1996

"I would give a lot to be where you are," was Fr. Michael's quiet response to my struggle. "Isn't this what you've been praying for—littleness, weakness, poverty, and humility? God has heard the deep cry of your heart. You've been praying to know your sins, and now you can stand in them and ask for mercy."

He told me not to be afraid of the anger and rebellion surging up within, but to let myself feel the emotions. He urged me to read the psalms.

October 3, 1996

Now that my back is better, I feel as if I have returned from a different country—a land of weakness, humiliation, and pain. Fr. Michael is right. This is precisely what I have been praying for. The Lord is leading me into a new spiritual reality, the reality of the cross, and I don't want to lose what I've been given.

October 8, 1996

From this morning's discussion with Marie, it looks as if I will be going to Combermere in March for a few months. My heart breaks at the thought of leaving Russia for so long and missing Lent and Easter here, but deep down, I know that my faith, and the reality of the cross in my life, cannot be bound even to Russia.

Working on the Russian edition of Catherine's autobiography, *Fragments of my Life*, I am struck as never before by her identification with the humiliated Christ. I too feel like a *yourodivyi*, a fool for Christ, as I beg God to continue what he is doing in me. Even as I weep, I ask him for more. What I want is life, life in abundance. *"Even though he slays me, yet will I trust."* (Job, 13:15)

All summer we pushed and pushed. The need was real, I tried to respond, and in the end, it was physically too much.

I ended up with bronchitis for six weeks, and I still have a sore back. But everything is part of his plan. God has used this sickness and incapacity to bring me to a new level of truth. As Jean once wrote in a newsletter, "Shoot me again, for I know I'm gonna live!"

October 15, 1996

Today I feel like an insect pinned to a board. Is this truly what the Lord wants for me? He allowed himself to be crucified and gave others power over him. Just as I was raging to myself, "This can't be a normal way to live!" I heard in my heart, "We're not talking about normality; we're talking about the Gospel."

Fr. Michael says I will only learn to accept the cross by learning to stand still in vulnerability and defencelessness.

"You must stop controlling," he said. "For you, it is absolutely imperative. If you don't crucify your mind, you will continue to live there, thinking it is reality. You will think you have moved to a new place, when all that has happened is that you have rearranged the furniture!

"The intellect limits, categorizes, and establishes boundaries," he continued. "The heart gives everything. Intellect is prudent and rationalizes. The heart is foolish and trusting."

"Unless you become like a little child, you will never enter the Kingdom of Heaven." (Mk 10:15)

Spiritual warfare

One day, our medic friend, Veronika's daughter Nelly, came to check on Marie and Alma, both of whom were recovering from a virus. I brought them tea in the bedroom and returned to the kitchen to have beans and rice with Misha (an English-speaking Buryat* friend), Lena, and her four-year-old son, Yaroslav.

Lena had appeared in the parish six months earlier. Small, wiry, always tense, with a thin face and pale eyes, she was usually wrapped in black from head to toe. After the murder of her Moslem husband in one of the Central Asian republics, Lena had fled with Yaroslav so

---

* Buryat – people of Mongolian origin, originally from Buryatia, a region adjacent to Irkutsk.

that her in-laws would not take him from her. Somehow, she ended up in Magadan. She was totally focused on obtaining what she and Yaroslav needed to survive. Nothing could divert her attention from this objective, and nothing else seemed to interest her. Each time she came to the house, we sensed a spiritual disturbance.

Miroslava arrived, and although she didn't usually stay when we had other guests, today she planted herself on a stool in the hall. When Misha left, Lena came out and struck up a conversation with Miroslava, somehow involving Nelly as well when the latter emerged from the bedroom. Nelly finally managed to extricate herself and left.

Lena began getting Yaroslav dressed to go home, always a time-consuming process. She continued to talk, and Yaroslav, who was roasting in his outdoor clothes, went to wait on the landing. While Lena made a phone call, I resumed visiting with Miroslava, who had now moved into the kitchen. I heard Lena hang up, went to say goodbye, and was engulfed in another stream of conversation. Left unsupervised, Miroslava darted into the bedroom to visit the sick.

It was three o'clock before I finally got Lena out the door and pried Miroslava away from Marie and Alma. The two of them were finally able to eat the lunch that had been sitting on a tray for two and a half hours. Miroslava accepted a cup of tea and she, too, left.

The doorbell rang again. It was Lena. She had lost Yaroslav, and she was frantic. He was not in the hall or on the stairs or in our courtyard or anywhere near the house. Even in the best of times, Lena was not one to reason calmly, and now she was both panic-stricken and hysterical.

No, she said categorically, the boy could not possibly have headed home by himself; he had never crossed the busy thoroughfare without her. However, she had seen Nelly looking at him strangely, and the only possible answer to Yaroslav's disappearance, she said, was that Nellie had kidnapped him.

We could hardly believe our ears, but nothing we could say would dislodge Lena's conviction. We finally let her phone Nelly in the hope that this might convince her, but Nelly's shocked denial had no effect.

I went out with Lena to look around once more, after which she returned to call the police. They told her to go home and wait.

Shortly afterward, a police car pulled up outside our building, and we watched from the window as Lena got in with them.

A little later Nelly phoned us in tears. The police and Lena had just been at her apartment, and Lena had again accused her of having kidnapped Yaroslav. We were appalled that Nelly, who had come as a friend to share with us her professional expertise, was now embroiled in this absurd situation. We could only imagine what it must mean to a Russian whose mother was a camp survivor to have the police come to her home on an accusation of kidnapping.

The phone rang all afternoon. I went alone to Mass, where fervent prayers were offered for the situation. When I returned home, Marie and Alma told me that Lena had called to say that Yaroslav had finally arrived, by himself, having spent time at a playground on the way.

After supper, we went into the chapel for a half hour of adoration. We were totally drained. Fr. Michael arrived towards the end and blessed us with the Blessed Sacrament. We stood around talking with him for a while longer; it was clear that the "baddies" had been out in force. Fr. Michael suggested that in such times of spiritual harassment, we lean on the spiritual protection of the priest. "You can deflect some of the attack my way," he told us.

The spiritual warfare was drawing us to an increasing intensity of prayer. Marie proposed that we extend our daily adoration to an hour. "It's the only weapon we have," she said.

November 12, 1996

My emotions are raging, and I can't use my mind to control them, as I've done for so long. Fr. Michael says to let the feelings surface and go, without attempting to sort things out. The circumstances themselves are not important. When attacked, I should stand in silence and feel the pain. This is how the heart becomes softened. Otherwise, he says, I will continue to analyze and rationalize my way around the cross. By standing in one's own pain, one learns to understand the pain of others.

When we get on to this theme, I find myself feeling like a pariah, "The Girl without a Heart." My mind, my best instrument, is suddenly my greatest obstacle.

November 19, 1996

In January I will turn fifty. Perhaps this is a good time to let go of what is not important. My good winter parka, for instance, which got ruined when I sat down on a bus seat where someone had accidentally dripped Chlorox.

God wants my life poured out in reparation. What does a parka matter? God is saying, "Don't get distracted. You have more important things to do. I am with you. Sit at my feet."

As a holocaust before the face of God

December brought Jean Fox, our beloved Director of Women, for a two-week visit. Shortly after her arrival, she went to bed with a terrible flu and dangerously high blood pressure. Although she eventually forced herself back on her feet, she never felt well and left exhausted. It was as if she had taken Magadan's spiritual warfare into her own body. She told us that as she lay so ill in our poustinia, she felt the presence and protection of Our Lady more powerfully than ever before in her life.

The bright side of the situation was that she was able to spend more time with us than if she had been able to accept other invitations. Once she began feeling well enough to be up during the day, we would return from Mass to find the laundry neatly folded and the dishes dried and put away. How wonderful it was to simply have her around!

One evening Jean joined us and some of our friends for the Wednesday rosary and tea. At her request, Alvina read the Russian translation of Catherine's story, "Russia on the Cross." I had hoped Jean might offer some reflections, but everyone started talking at once, and I had difficulty translating their comments for Jean. I did overhear Nadia say to Alvina, "I understood what you were reading. It is *because* we are on the cross that Russia will redeem the world."

Jean thought the story might have touched a raw nerve. "They are struggling to deal with the mystery of their own suffering," she said.

The day before she left Magadan, Jean spoke to us of what she had understood during her visit:

You need to stay very humble. Never think that through your own humanity, your own ideas, your own cleverness, or even your own charity, you will have an impact on anyone in Russia.

Have reverence for each person. Have reverence for their history and especially for the presence of God that is so tangible in each and every one of them. They are in a state of shock and are suffering grievously at this point in time. They are victims of history and of the tragedy that transpired in this country.

Let them wrestle with it themselves. Don't think you can teach them anything. Listen to them, love them, and embrace them as they themselves work out their return to faith. They will rediscover the face of Jesus Christ because Our Lady has promised.

Always keep in mind the purpose for which you are here: to love and serve your God, and to intercede and suffer and fast for the people of Russia. Many people can distribute material goods, *but very few can stand like a holocaust before the face of God, pleading for mercy.*

God is not interested in spiritual heroics, but in our love. Stand before him for the people. They themselves don't have the time. For them, we are the Church. We gather up their hearts and pour them back into the Blessed Sacrament.

Julia's baby

While Jean was ill, a strange episode occurred.

Alek Turkin had come into our life six months earlier, shortly after his release from prison where he had served a term for petty theft. He was trying to re-establish himself and would periodically stop by to visit. One day in October, while drinking with a woman acquaintance at her apartment, he had become angry at something. In his inebriated state, he struck the woman so hard that she fell, hitting her head on the corner of the iron radiator. She was taken, unconscious, to the hospital.

The following day, Alek came to use our telephone to check on the woman's condition. I was alone in the apartment and waited in the kitchen until I heard him hang up. When I went back into the hall, Alek's face was ashen. He fell into my arms, sobbing—not from grief, but from fear. The woman was dead, and Alek faced arrest for second-degree murder.

Terrified at the prospect of returning to prison, he fled somewhere up the Kolyma highway. We didn't want to know any more than that, in the event that we were questioned.

Toward the end of November, we received a visit from a girl in her late teens who introduced herself as Julia, Alek's long-term girlfriend and the mother of his eight-month-old son. She told us Alek had been arrested and was at the Magadan holding prison. She and the baby were staying with friends outside the city. Since the child was sick, we gave her money for medicine. Just before Jean's arrival in December, Julia returned with the news that the baby had been hospitalized.

On the night Jean fell ill, the doorbell rang at 1:30 A.M. We were all up quickly, thinking Jean might have come over from the poustinia. Instead we found Julia on the landing, sobbing.

"Little Alek is dead!" she wept.

Shocked and speechless, we drew her inside. Alma held her as the tragic story emerged. The baby had been in hospital with a high temperature, but had been doing better and was about to be discharged. Before Julia brought him home, the doctor insisted on one last I.V., administered through a vein in the head. A student nurse, assigned to prepare the treatment, mistakenly thought she was supposed to administer it as well. Within minutes the baby was dead.

It was a terrible story, but we had been in Magadan long enough to know it was all too plausible. We comforted Julia as we could, giving her tea and an herbal tranquilizer and putting her in Alma's bed. Alma pulled out a sleeping bag and slept in the chapel.

Julia spent the next few days with us. It was a hectic time, since we were caring for Jean and trying to keep everything else going as well, but we did our best to be present to Julia and to console her with our love. We bought her a ticket home, supplied her with food for the three-day trip, and saw her off at the bus station.

We didn't know how to contact Alek, but shortly after Julia's departure, he himself phoned from prison.

"Alek," Marie began, "I don't quite know how to tell you this... the baby is dead."

"What baby?"

"Your baby. Julia's baby."

Silence on the other end of the line. Then Alek said slowly, "She duped you. There is no baby. It was all a set-up."

We didn't begrudge Julia the money. But we had opened our hearts to her, holding nothing back, and her deception left a bitter taste.

Reorientation

On her return to Combermere, Jean wrote to us:

> My heart has been branded by Magadan. I offer my entire life as a holocaust for you and for the people there.
>
> We are deeply united. Fear nothing. Pray for the grace you need each day. Whatever happens is permitted by God for his glory. The Gospel is being incarnated there for all of Russia.
>
> Do not forget your weekly poustinias, and keep to your schedule as faithfully as you can. Work it out together and stick to it; this is crucial. We are being led by the Mother of God.
>
> Give my greetings to Fr. Michael and Fr. David. Convey my deep prayer, full of overwhelming tenderness, to the parishioners and all those who touched my heart so deeply with their love. Tell them they are icons of God himself. Tell them to rejoice in being crucified with the Saviour. He will resurrect all of Russia through their faith.

Behind Jean's admonition that we keep to a schedule, I sensed her concern for our health and a caution against excessive behaviour. Nevertheless, I was confused and dismayed. It was still such an ongoing struggle to respond to the poor, to serve without holding back—in short, to live the Gospel without compromise—that I didn't trust myself to draw limits. How could I hold back, just when I was learning to let go?

Marie received Jean's words as a directive to be carried out in unquestioning obedience. Perhaps it really was that simple. God asked one thing at one moment and at the next moment, something else. I had been called to let go completely and to give everything, and I had tried my best to respond. Now we were being called to pull back. Was it a matter of living the Gospel any less? It might not *feel* as if we were responding as wholeheartedly, I reasoned, but what mattered was that we not close our hearts.

It was becoming as evident to us as it had been to Jean that we couldn't continue responding as we had to the material needs of those who were coming to us. We had made it a point not to give money, but we found ourselves so busy trekking to the food stores to buy groceries for others that we could hardly do our own shopping! Our friends warned us that as North Americans, we were automatically considered wealthy and would be taken advantage of. Was this our call in Russia? Perhaps we needed the experience of being "used and abused," as Fr. Michael put it, to bring us to the humility of knowing we simply couldn't handle this type of apostolate.

"Many people can distribute material goods, but very few can stand like a holocaust before the face of God and plead for mercy." Jean's words had touched the essence.

Fortunately, Fr. Michael was quite willing for us to refer requests for food and clothing to him and to the parish program for humanitarian relief.

Alma heard it as a call to make prayer our priority. Trying to sort through the ambiguities in my own heart, I lacked her clarity.

"Why is it so painful?"
January 10, 1997

I am still pretty much in the same spiritual and emotional turmoil as when Jean was here.

Fr. Michael says that moving from the head to the heart is like letting go of one trapeze and being suspended in mid-air until you catch the next one. Faith is the belief that the second trapeze will be there for you.

He suggests that each time I feel hurt or offended, I fall to my knees (at least inwardly) and repent, without trying to determine who was right and who was wrong and without marshalling my defences and justifications. The publican at the back of the church didn't have a list of his sins; he only knew he was a sinner. In other words, stay at the back of the church and stand in the suffering, whatever form it takes. He told me not to fear the lack of clarity or the resulting anxiety, not to be afraid of tears or of strong, raw emotion. I have to learn to feel again, since thinking has become my defence against pain.

It sounds good and feels terrible.

January 17, 1997

I don't understand why the pain is so overwhelming; it is like being hit again and again in the same sore place. Like a little girl who keeps having her feelings hurt, all I want to do is cry.

Fr. Michael keeps telling me not to resist the pain, but to let God work.

"How long will it last?" I asked him.

"As long as God wants it. We don't pull from our suffering what is useful to us and then continue on our way. This is the beginning of a new life."

Poustinia, January 20, 1997

"Lord, why is it so painful?"
He pointed to the crucifix.
"Yes, but you suffered for us!"
"All suffering is united with my suffering."
"Are you sure these aren't just my neuroses?"
"I died for those too."

On the eve of my fiftieth birthday, I told God, *I will accept this pain as your will for me.*

The pain didn't diminish, at least not immediately, but I had crossed a threshold.

The following day, as I made an effort to respond to the love and good wishes that were being extended with obvious sincerity, something lifted. While there was no real change in the objective situation, it somehow seemed more bearable. It came to me that I had finally accepted love, not in the form I desired or thought I needed, but as it was offered.

When my back went out again on Ash Wednesday, I found myself on familiar ground. Once more, I struggled to surrender to the reality and to let go of all that I'd been planning to do. Ten days and a bottle of anti-inflammatories later, I was still no better.

I will lie here until you want me to get up, I said to God.

It was not an abstract surrender. It was a surrender to his love.

The same evening, Raissa, a retired medic versed in all sorts of healing and one of our more colourful acquaintances, appeared unexpectedly and offered to readjust my spine. Until now, I had resolutely resisted Raissa's treatments, but this time I decided to let her try. Marie was out. Alma was hovering in the background, poised to intervene the moment I gave the signal, but I wanted to see what would happen.

When I awoke the next morning, my back ached more painfully than ever, but it improved as the day progressed. Inexplicably, I felt enveloped in grace.

Fr. Michael later explained to me what he thought had taken place. Each time my back went out, he said, the sudden helplessness and physical pain forced me "out of my head and into my body." Unable to think myself out of the predicament, I would fall apart emotionally and flail around for support. By now, however, my supports had been pulled away. My only recourse was to accept the situation as God's will and surrender to it. Once I did this, in deep trust, without attempting to control even Raissa, I not only experienced spiritual healing, but I began to get better physically.

His analysis made deep sense to me.

February 28, 1997

This probably will be my last poustinia before I leave for Combermere.

Something definitive happened to me when my back was out, and I need to articulate it clearly so that it is stamped in my heart and in my consciousness:

I do not belong to myself, but to Christ. In pain, I experienced an intimacy with him that I could not find elsewhere. It isn't that I want the pain, or that I carry it well, *but I want you, Lord. My life is yours, to do with as you will. Please, give me the courage to follow your lead.*

Take Up Your Cross

This year's stay in Combermere changed my life.

Following a routine eye examination in April, the optometrist asked me to repeat a field vision test. The results showed damage to the optic nerve in the left eye, one cause of which could have been multiple sclerosis. Given my father's illness and my difficulty in walking, this seemed more than likely.

After a fall in the mid-1980s, I had suffered from lower back trouble, with attacks that became increasingly frequent. I was becoming more and more fatigued from the extensive walking we did in Magadan, and people often pointed out to me that I limped, but I attributed both conditions to my back problems. The possibility that they were linked to MS never entered my mind, since my family doctor had assured me that the disease was not hereditary.

Maureen, the community nurse, was away when I returned from the eye examination, and it was evening before I was able to see her. I was touched by her compassion. She thought the possibility of MS had to be taken seriously and explained that while the disease was not passed directly from one generation to another, there was still a genetic factor. "As I watched you walk," she said, "I was wondering about it myself."

All those to whom I was closest in Combermere were away, resting before the beginning of the Directors' Meetings. Marie had left Magadan and was somewhere in New England, visiting her niece. I was just as glad to have a few days in which to come to terms with the situation before sharing it with anyone.

My whole world had shifted.

Or had it?

As the initial shock subsided, it came to me that the possibility of having MS was strangely consistent with everything I'd been living, with everything God had been doing in my heart and in my life. With the rest of the Madonna House family, I had just renewed St. Louis de Monfort's consecration to Jesus through Mary, saying "I give myself to Jesus Christ...to carry my cross after him all the days of my life." During the pilgrimage to the camps, the cross had been planted even more firmly in my heart. Again and again throughout the year, the significance of the cross for my life had been reaffirmed, culminating in that moment of intimacy with Christ while my back was out.

God was inviting me to stand with him at the deepest level of my being and to offer him my life, in trust and surrender. If I did have MS, my years in Russia would be limited, but even the pain of this awareness was eclipsed by an overwhelming sense of God's presence and the revelation of his plan for my life.

I kept praying the de Monfort consecration and Charles de Foucauld's Prayer of Abandonment. My acceptance was not feigned, nor was the sense of being carried in an embrace of love. When Marie and other close friends arrived, I told them, and we cried together.

Then the medical rounds began: my doctor in Combermere, a neurologist in Ottawa, an ophthalmologist in Peterborough. The latter didn't think the eye problem was neurologically-related, but more likely a congenital condition or a low-pressure glaucoma.

Multiple sclerosis was usually diagnosed by Magnetic Resonance Imagery (MRI). Although in Canada, one usually needs to schedule MRIs months in advance, a new MRI department was being established at the Civic Hospital in Ottawa, and the neurologist arranged a scan for me even before it was officially open. This was quite extraordinary. And since he would be on holidays when the results reached his office, the neurologist agreed to my suggestion that I leave for Russia on the date I had originally planned, and that he forward the results to Combermere to be passed on to me. After all, I reasoned, even if I did have MS, the disease was incurable, so there wasn't much to do about it. Presumably, I would continue to live as before. Why wait around?

Marie and I had been planning to return to Russia together when the Directors' Meetings finished. I was looking forward to introducing her to my friends in Moscow and St. Petersburg, and I wanted to show her Fr. Men's parish. We were also planning to go to Latvia so that she could meet Fr. Viktor. I badly wanted to keep to our original schedule, and for once God indulged me: we left Combermere as planned at the end of May.

For both of us, the encounters with Fr. Viktor brought deep, deep blessing. The light emanating from him ignited our own hearts.

His joy and love and peace were so tangible that they made me desire the heavenly reality of which they were the fruit. Under his gaze of love, I felt as if my soul were light and smooth, and in his presence, I felt as free and happy as a child. Both Marie and I felt as if he knew us deeply.

When we said good-bye, I cupped my hands for his blessing, and he embraced me three times in honour of the Trinity. I began to weep, not from sentiment, but in response to a love different from any I had known.

Is it or isn't it?

Back in Magadan, five weeks had passed since the MRI, and I still hadn't received the results. I wanted to know, but strangely enough, I was not anxious about the diagnosis. The words that continued to resound in my heart were the ones I had received those first days, when the likelihood already seemed a fact: *my life belongs to God. It is his to do with as he wishes.*

This was not my usual approach to pain; normally, I economized my emotional energy until I knew what I had to contend with. This time, however, God was asking me to face the possibility, and all its spiritual implications, head-on. Whether or not I had MS, he was calling me to live at a point of abandonment. I was being plunged into the deepest reality of the spiritual life, and I didn't want to lose it, no matter what the diagnosis. Crazy as it seemed, God was using the possibility of this incurable disease to accomplish something absolute and irrevocable in my life.

If I did have MS, his plan would be clear. But if I didn't, how was I to live out what he was showing me? What came to me now was that I must take up the cross, deliberately and resolutely, in the context of daily living. This was pure Madonna House spirituality. Even if God was not calling me to give my life through a crippling illness, he was definitely calling me to offer my life day by day.

I didn't desire suffering, but I longed for the "desire to desire," so that, instead of evading pain, complaining about it, or even just enduring it, it might lead me to a union with Christ. To welcome all that happened to me as God's will was the key to peace—the kind of peace Fr. Viktor radiated.

June 27, 1997

Last Saturday I had a message to phone Combermere. When I did so, Maureen told me the MRI results had indicated that *I don't have MS.*

Paradoxically, what should have been good news threw me into a tailspin. All the pain and stress of the past two months has reopened, and I am left with a handicap for which I still have no explanation.

There wasn't time to do more than communicate the news to the others, as we were scheduled to go on a picnic with a whole group of people, including a visiting Japanese couple working with a humanitarian aid organization. Clinging to the arm of Lyuba's husband, I stumbled along over the uneven ground, and only later, while the others climbed down to the sea, was there a chance to let the tears spill forth.

It is humiliating to feel so utterly exposed, so vulnerable and defenceless. I would flee the emotions, but I know God is calling me to stand still.

Marie has suggested that I see our doctor friend for an orthopaedic workup. I hate getting involved in the medical merry-go-round here, but I have to do something. Whatever is wrong with me is getting worse.

July 4, 1997

To live a "camp spirituality" means to find life in the midst of death. The people in the camps left behind their talents, their creative potential, their initiative—everything. Perhaps our life in Magadan, with its particular frustrations, constitutes a way of reparation.

We can't feed all the hungry. It isn't for us to argue with those who are nostalgic for the ostensible securities of socialism. We can only come before the Blessed Sacrament, before the Lord *"who neither slumbers nor sleeps"* (Ps. 121) and intercede with our lives.

But how serious is my intercession? I asked myself this question yesterday, after Nina told us that when she was in Poland last month for the Eucharistic Congress, a member of the Magadan group was moved to renounce alcohol for a year, offering it for her son. "And I," Nina said, "gave it up for life for *my* son."

The uncalculated totality with which she moves leaves me breathless. Nothing is too much where Toli is concerned.

This is how I should be living!

July 11, 1997

Fr. Michael shared with us that, in poustinia, he had asked God how we might become one with the camp victims. The answer was, "Go to Our Lady. She will teach you. Our Lady was a victim."

"We don't *do* anything to become victims; we *receive* the Victim," he said. "We are not called to imitate Christ but to become Christ. We receive him in those who are victimized. Our hearts have to be empty so they can be open."

July 18, 1997

All day I've been trudging to doctors. The neurologist here told me that, on the basis of her clinical observations, I have MS. I tried to convey to her that I am not in denial, but that the most advanced medical technology in Canada has established that I don't have multiple sclerosis. I didn't know the Russian term for MRI, and she obviously isn't familiar with the procedure. She suggested that I be hospitalized here for observation and testing.

This kind of situation is more unbearable than a definitive diagnosis. Do I have it or don't I? How conclusive is the MRI? Should I go along with the medical procedures available here, or should I have further tests in Canada? What is God saying?

I have been reacting and over-reacting to everyone around me. Underlying the reactions is anxiety. Beneath the anxiety is fear.

Fr. Michael had some advice for me about how to live during this time of confusion and lack of clarity. He told me to plunge the spiritual thermometer down through the layers of my heart to the level from which the consecration to Our

Lady and our promises come. "Even if you don't feel it, do this as an act of the will."

At adoration Saturday night, in a moment of recklessness, I told God I wanted to be united with him as I have been in moments of suffering. I knew it was an imprudent move, but while my head said, "This is crazy," something deeper pushed me to go on.

August 30, 1997

I spent most of this week with Nina at her son's trial. It ended without a verdict. The evidence has to be sent to Khabarovsk for analysis by specialists; it could take up to a year, during which time the boys will continue to sit in jail. The prospect of a new trial, with everything repeated, is more than Nina can bear.

Nothing could ease the pain of that anticlimax. Tears streaming down her face, she asked me to walk with her for a bit. When she spoke, it was in a tiny, beaten voice. I hadn't understood a lot of what had gone on, and I didn't even catch all she was saying now, but I felt her pain pouring into my own heart.

All you who pass this way, look and see:
Is there any sorrow like the sorrow that afflicts me?
(Lam 1:12)

September 14, 1997 marked the fourth anniversary of our arrival in Magadan. The original team—Marie, Alma and myself—had been augmented by the arrival of Trudy Moessner the preceding March and in August, by Sushi Horwitz.

Four years ago none of us could have foreseen the breadth and depth of the spiritual life to which God would be calling us. Our first year had basically been one of acclimatization. The second had been marked by aridity, struggle, and spiritual battle. Fr. Michael had arrived, and I started spiritual direction with him. Once I began to fall in love with the Lord, I discovered the reality of my own sinfulness. I began learning how to stand in vulnerability, to renounce control, to recognize my fears. I met Our Lady and I began to desire the cross. Now God was permitting me to taste its reality.

In early November we finished our annual sauerkraut bee. After salting one hundred eighty-five kilos of cabbage (for ourselves and for Frs. Michael and David to share with needy parishioners), the next step was to relay thirty-five three-litre jars to the cellar. Still shaky after a bad fall a few days previously, I was terrified going down the steps with a heavy bottle in each arm.

The next day Sushi was in poustinia, and Marie and I were having lunch together in the kitchen. I felt weak and craved protein, but we'd given away the cheese, and there wasn't any peanut butter, and I didn't want to take the last egg. I settled on a second helping of seaweed. Since seaweed, though nutritious and even tasty when well prepared, had never been our most popular food option, Marie suspected something might be wrong. She boiled the egg for me, and we talked.

An hour later, the decision had been made that I should go to Combermere for further medical tests instead of trying to have them done here.

In poustinia, the following day, I sat by the window and watched the beautiful young women of Magadan lithely picking their way down the steep path and across the courtyard. In contrast, I saw myself stumbling down the street.

I cried and cried.

Grief? Self-pity?

A week later I went to the polyclinic to get the results of a blood analysis. The doctor told me my blood was normal. I was feeling so vulnerable, however, that I could barely control myself when she referred to "my MS" and told me about someone else who walked the same way I did. She was convinced that I was in denial.

Back home, everyone was rushing to get ready to go to Bronislava's seventieth birthday celebration. Marie and I left the house early, and as we were walking up Lenin Street, I mentioned how relieved I was that we'd decided against my going into the Magadan hospital for observation. I couldn't have handled it. But when I started to tell Marie about the doctor's comments, I suddenly found myself sobbing uncontrollably, right in the middle of the sidewalk. We retreated into a deep arch opening onto an inner courtyard, and I managed to pull myself together. Too unsteady to trust my balance, I had to hold Marie's arm for the rest of the way.

When I told Fr. Michael about the attack, he said there was a way to handle fear. "I'll show you," he promised, "but until then, pray for mercy. Mercy takes you beyond the cross and brings you before the face of God."

Later, at adoration, I said to Christ, *Right now, I can't even touch my heart through the fear, but I have already given my life to you many times. I claim that now, and I ask you to receive what has already been offered.*

November 18, 1997

Fr. Michael says I am standing in the center of my root struggle between fear and faith. One has to first acknowledge the emotion of fear and then turn from it to God. He says it is as if you are talking on the phone, and the doorbell rings. You say to the fear, "Excuse me, I have no time for you now. The King is here to see me."

When I described the inner pain and humiliation of my physical situation, he said I am standing squarely before the cross, and that on the other side is great freedom and the joy of intimacy with the Beloved.

Gratitude is the act that frees us. He told me not to force it, but to just make some movement of thanksgiving in my heart.

Yesterday I fell on the ice and spoke sharply when Marie and Sushi tried to pull me up too soon, before I'd had a chance to catch my breath. Then I realized it wasn't Marie and Sushi helping me, but a Russian man. At my reaction, he quickly walked away. Sushi and Marie accompanied me home in silence, while I fought tears. We all slip on the ice, but for me, it brings home the reality of this handicap—disease—whatever it is I have.

December 19, 1997

All year we've been talking about intimacy with God in suffering. The thought is as repulsive as ever—and as sweet. I am still afraid of pain, yet I have experienced intimacy with the Lord in those very moments, and I know this is the source of a life I can barely imagine.

There is no way I can embrace suffering with my mind. I can only keep moving from my heart—from the place where I say to God, "I love you," without analyzing, reflecting, or weighing the possible consequences of my words. My heart says, "I love you," without considering whether or not the words can be lived out. The heart is an utterly reckless organ and totally gullible—it believes that whatever comes from it is truth!

My heart says, "Lord, I embrace your cross in love and trust, in gratitude and adoration. I want to be with you. I want to know you as I knew you that time when my back was out, and when I thought I had MS. I know there is no other way but through the cross. I accept your conditions. I accept them for myself so that I may know you, and I accept them for the sake of all our friends in Magadan, for Russia, for Madonna House, for the Church of East and West."

February 1998

Back in Combermere I sat down with Maureen, and we drew up a plan to track down the cause of my walking difficulties. Anxiety came and went. I returned to the specialist I'd seen the year before. He did a simple neurological examination and, to my immense relief, said he would arrange for me to be admitted to the Ottawa General Hospital for further testing.

The morning after my admission to the hospital, I was given another MRI. By mid-afternoon the results were clear.

"You have multiple sclerosis," the doctor told me.

Unbelievably, since I'd known for almost a year that this was the most plausible diagnosis, I was caught off guard. I had brought a stack of books and my embroidery to keep me occupied while undergoing a battery of diagnostic tests, and a wad of money in case I was allowed to leave the hospital on the weekend. I hadn't thought twice about taking a large amount of cash, as we did it all the time in Russia, but the nurses on the neurology floor were horrified and made me put the money in a safety deposit box. With all these distractions, I had momentarily forgotten how much was at stake.

My mind reeled with the finality of the verdict.

The doctor said I could go home. I phoned Madonna House. It would take Maureen at least two and a half hours to drive in from Combermere to bring me back. In the meantime I went down to the main floor of the hospital to retrieve the money I'd locked away only twenty-four hours earlier. I was in a fog, fighting to control the flood of emotions surging within. I took my money from the safety deposit box and returned the key to the administration desk. As I turned to enter the elevator, I saw a sign that read "Chapel" and moved blindly in that direction.

I had expected it to be an interdenominational prayer room, but to my surprise, the Blessed Sacrament was there. It was as if God himself were waiting for me. As I sank to my knees, I heard in my heart, *"I am giving you the gift you wanted. Now you will be united with me forever."*

Maureen arrived at the hospital in record time. Walking into my room, she took me in her arms. I sobbed a little, but beneath the tears was acceptance—the fruit of God's words to me in the chapel. Maureen took me out for a lobster dinner with plenty of wine and responded to my questions about MS with a directness I appreciated.

We spent the night in Ottawa at a residence run by nuns and drove home the next morning. No sooner had we turned into the Madonna House yard than we spotted Jean coming toward us. Jumping out of the car to embrace her, I saw tears in her eyes. Maureen slid out from behind the steering wheel so that Jean could slide in. We drove to the building where I was staying, and I told her everything.

When I spoke of what had happened in the hospital chapel, her eyes once more filled with tears. "Miriam," she said, "you've given him everything. You've given him your mind, you've given him your emotions, and now you've given him your body. He will be faithful to you."

I felt her love, her care, her compassion. And her pain.

Picking up the cross

As the airplane landed in Magadan, I leaned my head against the window and wept.

Everything seemed beautiful to me—the shabby little airport, ugly Proletarskaya Street, our apartment building with its peeling paint and graffiti on the door. The cold, crisp air and the blue northern sky. The familiar stairs and our apartment that always seemed so small and cluttered for the first moments after a long absence. Home!

Marie had given me the most "private" bed in our dormitory-office. Covering it was a new blanket, so soft and thick that I felt warm just looking at it. She showed me the letter she had received from Jean:

> Miriam is definitely going to have limitations. She has to have adequate rest, and this means naps, early bedtime, and listening to her body. Heroic asceticism on the physical level is *not* God's will for her. Encourage her to take the bus to church, whenever she can.

When Jean had spoken of this in Combermere, I had felt as if a sword were being thrust into my heart. I didn't want to change my life—I loved our life! I loved the spiritual challenge of being drawn beyond my perceived limits; I wanted to keep giving myself, but Jean said that God's will for me now was to invest my energy in the Russian publications—"not to become crippled in two years!"

"I'm not telling you to take care of *yourself*," she clarified. "That would indeed be awful. I'm telling you to take care of your *body*."

Though far from serene, I felt no revolt. Grief, yes, along with anxiety, self-will, and confusion. Everyone would have understood, had I cried out, "I don't *want* to have MS," but even deeper than the grief lay acceptance. The deepest reality of my life was spiritual. I'd come too far to reject the cross now.

Fr. Michael began to open for me the Little Way of St. Therese of Lisieux, the essence of which consisted in offering to God as a sacrifice absolutely everything that happened in one's life. For example, when I voiced my reluctance to take care of myself in ways our friends couldn't, he said firmly, "You turn it all back to God, exactly as Therese did, keeping nothing for yourself. Offer your rest as a sacrifice for those who can't rest. Take medication for the sake of those who can't afford medication. You do everything out of obedience. This is the way suffering becomes intercession."

Tears sprang to my eyes. "I was so afraid you wouldn't understand. I was afraid I'd be cut off from what everyone else is living. I'm so grateful!"

March 31, 1998

At one time in my life, I would have considered myself fortunate to be able to sleep in each morning, rest after lunch, and excuse myself at 9 P.M. Why do I now feel as if I'm being held in a straightjacket?

"You've lost your freedom," was Marie's explanation. Then she added that perhaps I have lost one freedom only to find another. What came to me later was the phrase, "You are in bondage to the cross."

Yes, the loss of freedom is bitter. I am not allowed to live the disease as I choose. I'm not free to ignore my fatigue or to fast—in fact, I'm no longer able to fast in a physical way; my body won't tolerate hunger.

How could I suddenly have become so much weaker? Before going to Combermere, I was walking to church and back each day, and now I feel wiped out if I walk even one way. Marie says it's because I've given myself permission to feel fatigue.

I don't like it, but I've no other choice.

I am the bond servant of the Lord. The bond servant of Our Lady.

"Whither thou goest, I will go."

Wednesday of Holy Week, April 8, 1998

Yesterday we made *koolitch,* the traditional Russian Easter bread. To be exact, the others made it; I was in poustinia. And since everyone's energy and time are at a premium, Marie has decided to bake less this year and to serve it here to our guests instead of giving it away, as we've done in the past.

I find this so painful—it's bad enough that I can't participate myself, but I don't want anything more to change! I don't want to lose the familiar world around me!

When we talked about it later, Marie said something astonishing. For many years, I had assumed that a person with
a serious illness was an extra burden for an active field house
to carry. I had taken it for granted that, in order to remain in
Magadan, I would have to live my infirmity as unobtrusively
as possible so that it did not interfere with the community
life. But instead of my illness being an impediment to our
apostolate, Marie sees it as an instrument God is using to
point us all in a new direction. He is calling us to become
holocausts and, at the same time, to let go of activities that
have become less essential—like baking *koolitch* to give away.
Many of the things that pressure us, she said, are actually of
our own making.

What Marie was now saying reminded me of Raia and
Volodya's reaction when Raia's daughter became pregnant:
"We will not pretend it didn't happen. Let our lives change!
We will accept this child and love it. We will give our lives in
love and support."

Oh, you Russian hearts, you *Christian* hearts! How blessed
we are that our own hearts are being opened by the lance of
suffering! We are one; our lives cannot be separated. We are
called to give our lives for each other, and together, we have
to let them shift. God's will is revealed through events, and
we respond *together*. This is more obvious to Russians than to
us, individualistic Americans that we are. I myself am barely
beginning to perceive it.

The goal of this *podvig*, this spiritual adventure, must be
love and compassion; otherwise it is wasted. I had just a
taste of it the other night, returning from Mass on the bus
with Daria, one of the poorest of the poor, while the others
walked home. I was in such inner pain that all I could do
was to let it flow out in tenderness toward Daria. For just an
instant, I stood in the right position of the heart.

On Good Friday, I tripped and fell on the way to the church
services. How appropriate, I thought ruefully, brushing the snow
from my coat. It had been a day without human consolation, but the
liturgy swept away everything except the reality of Christ's sacrifice.

Afterwards, when everyone else had left the chapel, I knelt before the Blessed Sacrament and, with Fr. Michael and Marie as witnesses, consecrated my MS to Christ in words that had come to me in the poustinia:

> This illness is like a covenant. *"I have given you the gift you wanted. Now you are united with me forever."*
>
> It is the seal of love in my flesh. God has given me this illness in his mercy because he knows my weakness, and he knows the desire of my heart. I can no longer escape from him from whom I don't want to escape. Even my sins won't keep me from him. I who run from the cross am now bound to it with bonds of love. I, who so instinctively clutch for support, am forced to stand with Christ in the aloneness none but he can share.
>
> Now I want to ratify my side of this covenant. I want to consecrate to God my illness of multiple sclerosis. I accept it with all my heart, and I offer it in atonement for those who suffered in the camps of Kolyma and other places in Russia. I offer it in reparation and for an end to the evil and suffering perpetrated in this country. I offer it for the purification and sanctification of the Catholic and Orthodox Churches in Russia. I offer it for the protection and sanctification of our little parish in Magadan. I offer it for the priests of this country and especially for our priests here—for Fr. Michael and Fr. David. I offer it for all of Madonna House.

That was a lot for one little person, but by now, I was less afraid of aiming high. There was no way I could live out those words by my own efforts. But I had come to believe that with grace, all was possible and that living by the Spirit was quite different from spiritualizing. Despite the fear that still inhabited me, I could proclaim those words because they were guaranteed by God's own fidelity.

"One with them, one with me"

During the Easter Sunday liturgy, one of the parishioners turned and started to make a scene. I never did find out what had occasioned the outburst, but Nina, who was sitting next to the person, remarked later, "People are living with so much stress and so many insoluble problems that they reach a point where they can't take any more, and then they explode. After that they can go on."

The same sense of hopelessness erupted around our Easter dinner table that evening. When the other guests had departed, Fr. Michael observed quietly, "The situation here in Russia is literally driving people crazy. There is nothing we can do to fix it. The only thing we can do for them is to become holocausts."

It had been months since those on the government payroll, including medical personnel and teachers, had received their salaries. Polina came to beg money, not for herself, but for our mutual friend Larissa, with whom Polina teaches at the High School of the Arts. Larissa is in the hospital awaiting surgery, but the doctors will not operate until she purchases the medicines she will need.

"We work like slaves, without pay, and we have to beg for antibiotics!" Polina said with tears in her eyes. "I didn't want to come to you, but there is no one else who can help. You are the only ones who have money!"

And *I* complained about feeling humiliated!

After hearing Bronislava and Olga, another elderly camp survivor with whom we had become close, talk about the hunger in the camps, we no longer use the phrase, "I'm starving." Having seen the ice cells at the gulag site, we vowed to no longer complain about the cold. In the same way, I needed to offer my own little pricks of humiliation for Polina, Larissa, and all the others.

Easter Saturday, April 18, 1998

I asked Fr. Michael how one offers pain.

He answered, "Accept it. Feel it. Offer it to Christ."

When I told him I was afraid the MS would affect my mind, he prayed for a moment and said, "Give your life to God in this moment. Offer up this moment. Anything that takes you out of the moment is a temptation."

I understand that it is important to learn to live from my heart *now*. My legs may go. My eyes may go. My mind may go. If my treasure is my mind, I'm dead, but if I am living from the heart, I will be fully alive.

Alma's transfer to Combermere that June, after five years in Magadan, occasioned an immense outpouring of love from our friends, who ranged from our eleven-year-old neighbour Anyusha to seventy-year-old Bronislava. Although the Russian language had been an ongoing crucifixion for Alma, her big-hearted generosity and unstinted self-giving had borne more fruit than any degree of linguistic achievement.

People came for days to say goodbye and to bring gifts. Tanya and her son Kirill must have paid six visits. Our librarian friends came for an evening. As they were leaving, Alma and the four librarians hugged each other warmly; then they stood and talked some more. Another round of hugs. Only after the fourth exchange of embraces did the librarians finally take their leave!

The night of Alma's departure, we called a taxi to take her to the airport. Marie accompanied her, and Trudy and I stood outside with a group of friends, waving good-bye. I felt I was seeing the end of the foundational phase of this house.

July 7, 1998

With Alma gone, we are again short-handed. Everyone is overworked, and I am not the only one suffering from fatigue. When I asked Marie if the priorities established for me last spring were still valid under these new circumstances, her response was affirmative and emphatic. What is more, she suggested I begin working and resting in the kitchen of the poustinia apartment, away from the house activity. Although it increases my sense of isolation and exacerbates the loneliness, she considers it an organic part of my call to a more contemplative role in the community. She feels I will lead the house into that focus. But for me, it is a walk in pure faith.

July 17, 1998

Today on TV we watched with mixed feelings the state burial of the remains of Tsar Nicholas II and his family in the chapel of the Peter and Paul Fortress in St. Petersburg. One wanted to believe that this event was, indeed, as historic as it might seem: a complete reversal of the past seventy years, an acknowledgment by the entire society that a sin had been committed.

However, it wasn't "the entire society" that was burying the Imperial Family; it wasn't even clear who *was* backing this event. As always, the Romanov family was divided and its factions were quarrelling among themselves. President Yeltsin only decided to attend at the last minute, and the Russian Orthodox patriarchate distanced itself from the ceremony to such an extent that they would not permit the names of the Tsar and his family to be mentioned in the prayers. The patriarchate claims there is insufficient evidence to establish the authenticity of the remains. This is important, because if the Imperial Family is canonized, as seems probable, their bones will become objects of veneration.

Needless to say, nobody repented or atoned for anything.

When I asked a few of our friends about their impressions, the answers ranged from scepticism to indifference. Our friends are, for the most part, products of the Soviet educational system.

Just the same, we are left with a sense of awe. What has taken place would have been inconceivable even eight years ago, and it only seems right that the souls of the murdered Romanovs have been brought to rest in the prayer of the Church.

July 22, 1998

I hate to think about how I look when I walk, legs wobbling, out of control. I am now one of the poor. *Lord, help me to see it as a grace. You, who were "so disfigured that [you] seemed no longer human" (Is 52:14), show me the mystery of the poor, the disfigured, the "goners"—those who were dying of starvation in the camps and who had lost all but a semblance of their humanity.*

The fear, the uncertainty, the humiliation, the loneliness and limitations are all part of what I have chosen to embrace. When I remember this, the grace of God's gift—of the covenant—bursts forth to cover and free me.

Yesterday, as I stood waiting for the bus, a grandmother gave me an apple!

August 31, 1998

At times I feel as if my body were a time bomb waiting to explode. I am tempted to gobble up life while I am still mobile. I want to drink up the summer sun and the beauty at the *dacha** while I can still get out there. But I am called to live in the present moment, rather than store up for the future. One of the words that came to me recently, in the midst of the pain, was, *"I want to use this time to prepare your heart."*

Why then do I cry so uncontrollably? Why does it feel as if my heart is being sucked right out of me? If Marie had not invited me to talk the other day, would I have been able to stand in the pain until it brought me before him whom my heart loves?

The crises of 1998

On August 17, 1998, the Russian rouble was devaluated, and the country defaulted on its foreign debts. One day in September, the exchange rate for the dollar rose to twenty-eight roubles, falling the next day to fifteen. Banks were closed and prices on food commodities doubled. People began panic-buying. Warehouses closed until merchandise could be re-priced, leaving store shelves un-replenished.

The prime minister had been fired. Word got out that the pension funds were empty and that from now on, hospital patients would have to bring their own food. There were rumours about food shortages and lack of coal for the coming winter. Teachers were told not to expect their salaries, but to keep on working! As usual, the hot water had been shut off in August so that the system could be cleaned; now we heard that it wouldn't be turned back on until November first. In the villages on the Kolyma highway, conditions were said to be critical.

We watched TV in an attempt to understand what was transpiring, but the news clips of ministerial meetings and their endless discussions of high finance seemed unrelated to the anger and despera-

---

* *Dacha:* a summer cottage with a garden; in our case, a two-room shack.

tion we encountered each day. A routine, "How are you?" elicited a growled, "How *can* one be in a country like this?"

It seemed to me that the crisis was not only political and economic, but also spiritual. The fundamental vacuum left by communism was being exposed. Money and sleek, materialistic Westernization had become reigning deities, and their failure had led the country to ruin.

"There is no God but you, O Lord."

On October seventh, the feast of the Rosary, I came out of poustinia and found Marie talking on the phone with Fr. Michael. The call went on and on, and the tone sounded ominous. When she finally hung up, Marie said that Fr. Michael's visa was being re-examined in conjunction with a new law concerning religious organizations. The situation was extremely serious.

A little later Fr. Michael himself appeared at the door. He was visibly shaken. After joining us for adoration of the Blessed Sacrament, he recounted the whole story, including the possibility he might have to leave the country in three weeks. It was not at all certain he would be readmitted. In that case Fr. David's time in Magadan would also be limited, and the parish might conceivably find itself without a priest.

Bishop Werth was away from Russia and couldn't be reached. Fr. Michael had spoken with our new auxiliary bishop, Jerzy* Mazur, by phone, but although the latter was supportive, he was too new to be of practical assistance.

In my heart I heard, *"Offer yourself."*

"Oh, I do!" I cried silently.

My secret weapon was not just my body; it was my whole life. Even if it meant I had to be the one to leave Russia, I couldn't hold anything back. I finally understood that to be a victim soul meant to sacrifice oneself out of love.

"A man can have no greater love than to lay down his life for his friend." (Jn 15:13)

"The Father loves me because I lay down my life in order to take it up again. No one takes it from me; I lay it down of my own free will." (Jn 10: 17–18)

---

* Pronounced "YE-zhy".

October 22, 1998

In the course of these stress-filled and prayer-filled weeks, God has been teaching me not to pay too much attention to how I feel. I am learning to thank him when I feel poorly and when I feel well. The point is not how one feels, but to offer everything.

This illness is God's will for me. Oh, the pain will come again, along with the desire to be able to just put on my coat and walk out the door, like everyone else. But acceptance is there: fragile, yet real.

I have finally realized what it is that has been so hard to grasp since I received this diagnosis. For most of our time in Magadan, we have bent our wills to go further and further in living the Gospel. Suddenly, it seemed I was being asked to do the opposite, to let my body dictate the choices and to *not* will to go beyond my physical limitations. Now I see that the first instance involves the use of my will and the second, embracing God's will. When I do so, his grace does the work for me. St. Therese describes it as using a lift, instead of trying to pull oneself up the staircase by one's own efforts.

Marie feels that this is the direction in which we are all being called.

Madonna House Magadan Newsletter

November 7, 1998

Dear Family,

The economic and political crisis that struck Russia in mid-August is still far from having been resolved. Though the situation is somewhat calmer now, its effects continue in the lives of our friends—lives that already seemed stretched almost to the breaking point.

We've never understood how people who haven't been paid in months continue to feed their families, and now, prices have doubled! Some of our teacher friends recently received the salary that had been due in March, only to discover that it was worth less than half its original buying power. One woman, who had been waiting to send money to her son in Ukraine, burst into tears when she realized how little the roubles are worth since the devaluation. Another friend has been putting money into a bank account in preparation for moving to St. Petersburg. The bank has closed, and her savings are lost.

People dream of leaving Russia for another country—any country where they might be able to live a normal life—but most of them have to just stay and cope as they can. Our Orthodox bishop told Fr. Michael, "It was worse in the past." But people had been hoping it would be better.

Since the beginning of September, we have received little overseas mail. From what we are able to understand, the airlines are refusing to carry it because the money earmarked for this service by the government has been frozen in the banks.

The city has only a third of the coal needed for the winter, and at this point, the heating is so minimal that one hardly notices it has been turned on.* Now, as the real cold sets in, we are relying on electric heaters. No one knows what will happen next.

Ironically, it was just when we were wondering if we would be allowed to stay in Russia at all that the owner of the two-room apartment across the landing announced she was ready to sell—and we bought our third apartment! It will be used for poustinias and a publications office.

I want to thank all of you for your love and prayers following my MS diagnosis last March. I am doing well. I am so grateful to be here in Magadan, and I am learning, day by day, how to offer this illness for the people and the Church of this country. It is a new way of life, but it is part of the mystery in which God is calling us to live here in Russia.

In Our Lady of Magadan,
Miriam for all

---

* The heat for the whole city was controlled from a central heating plant.

November 18, 1998

Yesterday I sat in the kitchen talking to Lyuda Yaretik, my back to the window. I could feel the room getting colder and colder, but I didn't want to break off the conversation to turn around. With the radiators barely warm to the touch, we have been using the electric oven to warm the kitchen, and I hadn't realized that Trudy had turned it off. Lyuda, not having removed her coat, didn't notice the difference. By the time she left, though, my legs were rigid and my feet felt like blocks of ice. Even with a hot water bottle, and the electric heater turned up as far as it would go, it took me a couple hours to thaw out.

Thinking of the ice cells didn't help this time—I can't even imagine that magnitude of suffering!

December 1, 1998

My nightly leg spasms are getting worse and more continuous. Marie is worried about how the cold affects the MS and is wondering if I should go to Combermere right after New Year's. Much as I too have been dreading the cold, I dread even more the thought of being separated from everything here that gives me the courage to go on.

Friends have been coming to the house and bursting into tears. For them, we are an inn of the heart.

People are becoming ill from unheated rooms. What about babies, the elderly, the sick? University students and professors are wearing coats, boots, and heavy mitts in the classroom. Elementary schools are freezing cold. At first the younger children were sent home, but since all their mothers worked, the children found themselves alone in their chilly apartments. Our friend Tanya went around to the homes of her first grade pupils to be sure they were all right.

Week after week, Frs. Michael and David are calling people to a deeper level of hope. As Fr. Michael said so movingly last Sunday, "Suffering opens our hearts, and when our hearts are open, *God always comes*."

This Advent will truly be one of waiting, longing, and expectation.

One evening, as we were discussing the crisis situation in the city, Marie turned to Trudy and asked, "If things get worse, do you want to stay?"

"I wouldn't miss it for the world," Trudy answered with a weak smile.

She didn't ask me! And understandably, for even at this point, my muscles were stiffening in the cold and going into spasms. I wanted to burst into tears.

"To have to leave is also giving your life," Fr. Michael told me later. He added, "It is important for us that you do this." I should have been consoled, but the implication that I was no longer part of "us" was a sword in my heart.

A few days later, we were sitting around the kitchen table and suddenly realized the apartment was warmer! The heat in the radiators had increased just enough that it no long required a major effort to leave the warmth of the electric heater and go out into the hall.

The intense cold spell had also broken. I shed a layer of clothing, returned to house slippers from the felt boots I'd been wearing, and was able to move around the apartment again without my leg muscles contracting. Coal was supposedly on its way.

Even while I seemed to have been given a reprieve, I was coming to understand that my terror at the possibility of having to leave Magadan was alienating me from God.

"I can't let go," I said to Fr. Michael.

"Miriam, you must," he answered. "Otherwise, everything you offer will turn to ashes. It will be covered with self and encrusted with fear. But you can't do it by yourself. Pray for the grace. The opposite of fear is trust."

In mid-January I left for medical appointments in Combermere. I had reserved a return ticket for two months later, but Jean felt I should stay until after Easter to rest and adjust to medication. This was the last thing I wanted to do! When I phoned Magadan to tell them, Fr. Michael happened to be visiting and came to the telephone. He said, "God is breaking your will because it is strong, and your mind, which loves to plan. He is asking you to take what is most precious to you and offer it to him. He wants to be your sole delight."

As his words broke through my rebellion, what had seemed a sentence of exile became an invitation. I was staying on in Combermere because the *Lord* wished it!

Letter to Miriam from Fr. Michael Shields

March 5, 1999

My dear sister,

I read and prayed with your letter, and I feel the struggle with your will. Miriam, it is all about death. You just have to keep reminding yourself that nothing is yours now. All is your Beloved's. Your body is not yours, your will is not yours, your future is not yours, your life is not yours. Nothing is yours. This is truly the struggle.

You, dear friend, have to remember that nothing is yours. When you do remember this, I see the freedom and joy bubbling up within you. When you have nothing, then you have nothing to lose and therefore, nothing to fear and nothing to fight for. You are free to love where you are and to be poor, little, and an instrument of mercy for others.

I see death as the key to this struggle. Miriam, you are going to die one way or another, so run into the arms of Jesus, giving him everything and asking nothing for yourself. There is no other way for you. You are on the cross, but it is your joy. Let death become your way of life, and let your heart sing each day, "I am closer to him for whom my heart longs! Take my body and my will and all my fears; I want nothing else but him and him alone in my heart." Nothing else will satisfy your hunger now, and any temptation to hold on to future, past, or self will just make you more confused and anxious. Letting go of future, past, and self will bring you peace and complete joy.

So, my dear friend with whom I suffer, let's simply die now, today. Give it all up; there is no use in fighting. He has your heart and you are his. Let him love you in death, and therefore, live for him now and forever. I know this is all you want.

I am with you in prayer, and I know he has you in the care of his mother—what better company can there be?

Die here, die there, JUST DIE! And remember—we have all we need to be crucified. Isn't it great?

Love,
Fr. Michael of the Heart of Jesus.

Dom Madonny / Madonna House

Proletarskaya St, No. 46/2 – 2nd Floor

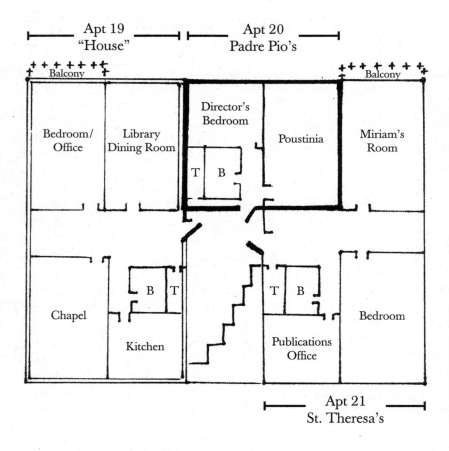

Follow Me

Madonna House Magadan Newsletter
from Trudy Moessner

April 11, 1999

Dear Madonna House Family,

I've just come from Mass to the church office to write this long overdue newsletter so that Marie can bring it to Combermere when she flies out four days from now.

Today is Easter Sunday in Russia, the second one, and we join our hearts and prayers with our Orthodox brothers and sisters as they celebrate the Lord's resurrection. For the second consecutive Sunday, a table was set up in our church for the blessing of Easter eggs and *koolitch.* After the long, hard winter, this Easter is a source of hope and joy for those who have been living with such heavy burdens.

In our midst right now is one of the greatest missionaries of all time—the small relics of St. Therese of Lisieux are with us for ten days. She is on pilgrimage through Russia, and the entire parish is praying a novena to her. May she who wanted to spend her heaven doing good on earth truly bless this far corner of our diocese!

Fr. Michael has been instrumental in arranging her journey through Siberia. In a few days, he will leave to meet her large reliquary and accompany it to Irkutsk. Fr. David, Sushi, and I will fly to meet him there and join the rest of the diocesan workers for a pastoral conference—the first "gathering of the clan" since the formation of this new diocese of Irkutsk.* We know the Little Flower's presence will be a tremendous grace for us all.

---

* Technically, Irkutsk was still part of the Apostolic Administration of Asiatic Russia, but Bishop Mazur had been given *de facto* responsibility for the eastern half of this vast region. In 2002 the two apostolic administrations in the Russian Republic were officially divided and erected into four dioceses.

We will have to fly to Moscow in order to make the return connection to Magadan. It is roughly comparable to flying from Pittsburgh to Los Angeles in order to get to Boston!
We are hoping to meet up with our long-awaited Miriam in
the Moscow airport and fly back home together.

Last week we finally received the keys to our new two-
room apartment, which we bought from our neighbour last
winter. A work crew has already begun to tear down three
layers of wallpaper, paint the ceilings, and do other needed
renovations. Miriam will have her room there, as well as an
office in which to work on the publication of Catherine's
writings in Russian.

Christ is risen! Truly he is risen!
Let us rejoice in his victory! Let us live in his love!

Trudy, for Marie, Sushi, and Miriam
(in Combermere)

MAGADAN

Before leaving Combermere for Magadan, I had a long talk with
Marie, who had just arrived for the Directors' Meetings. She suggested I spend two days in poustinia, once the third apartment was
ready. God had moved me into a new spiritual space, she said, and
I needed a way of life that would enable me to keep standing before him in surrender and trust. Both Marie and Jean warned me
against the temptation of becoming involved in the daily running of
the house.

I was relieved by the neurologist's observation that, apart from
some weakening in my legs, the disease had not progressed. After
the prolonged rest in Combermere and with new medication, I was
actually feeling much better. I had less pain and less fatigue and was
sleeping, if not soundly, at least through the night.

Toli

Several weeks after our return to Magadan, Nina's twenty-three-
year-old son, Toli, was sentenced to eight years at a prison camp

for rape, notwithstanding the fact that the girl had withdrawn her accusation. Everyone was stunned at the severity of the sentence, especially at this time when prisoners were known to be suffering acutely from hunger and cold.

The trial had ended more quickly than anyone expected, and neither Nina nor Nadia, her half-sister, was present to hear the verdict. Nadia phoned us from the music school as soon as she got the news, then rushed off to the courthouse to see her nephew before he was taken away. Nina had already left the school and had just arrived home when a neighbour gave her the message. She ran back out to the street, caught a taxi, and got to the courthouse just in time to meet her son's eyes as he was herded into the prison van.

I was tempted to hobble over to the courthouse to join them, but I had already used up my energy for the day. Besides, something in me said, "Let people come to *you*." I wandered about the apartment, unable to concentrate on anything until little Lenochka, Nadia's granddaughter, came running up the stairs to say that Nina and Nadia were on their way. I had been right to stay in the house of Our Lady so that they might come to her for solace.

Trudy was out doing errands, and Sushi was next door in the poustinia. I asked Lenochka to fetch her. When the others arrived, we went straight to the chapel and fell to our knees. Nina broke down, sobbing uncontrollably. I sat next to her, helplessly; there was nothing, absolutely nothing I could do or say. After a while I stroked her back. For years they had been praying for Toli's acquittal; what could prayer mean to them now? Finally we said a decade of the rosary for his strength and courage, and they left in silence.

Another beginning

July 13, 1999

Marie returned a few days ago, accompanied by Catherine Lesage, whom we are calling by her Russian diminutive, Katia. She will be with us from now on.

Janet Bourdet is also here, on loan from Madonna House in Arizona to present the Montessori "Catechesis of the Good Shepherd" at the parish summer school. One of the teenagers, Kira, will be her translator.

As usual, the changed dynamics in the house, not to mention the move to the third apartment, have me clutching to find a foothold on life. I feel stripped of everything familiar, buried alive in this new, cold, beautiful room and set apart from the daily flow of the community. It's as if my life has been taken away from me. I know this isn't true, and I know the things I grieve for are insignificant, but up to now, they have made up the fabric of my Magadan existence.

I am being freed from house duties in order to pray, rest, and work on the Russian publications. Why is it so painful to no longer be carrying responsibility in the house? Gnawing at me is the fear I am no longer capable of exercising leadership. I have difficulty in thinking abstractly and in keeping the broader picture in my mind. Fatigue and the need to always pace myself means I can no longer participate in community life as I did before.

This is the *kenosis** into which multiple sclerosis has thrust me. It is an essential aspect of the poustinia vocation, but nobody asked me if I wanted it! No, that's not true. God asked me, and I said yes, and now I must let go of one life in order to grow in another.

I meet him on the marriage bed of the cross.

June 15, 1999

Fr. Michael told me, "On the path where God is leading you, you have to stop depending on relationships."

This no longer terrifies me as it used to. "Resistance" would better describe my attitude. But last night, the thought that momentarily broke through the pain was, "All this has to be cut away, so that he can fill you with himself." I need to focus not on the stripping, but on the filling.

When the tears welled up once more, I asked God to protect me from temptation. I said the prayer of abandonment, the consecration to Our Lady, and the consecration of my MS. I said them with my will, as an act of faith, choos-

---

* *Kenosis* (Gr.)— interior emptying so that we might be filled with Christ. See Ch. 12, "Kenosis", in *Poustinia* by Catherine Doherty, Madonna House Publications, 2000, pp. 111–121.

ing with my will God's will for me. This is all I can do right
now.

July 20, 1999

I was up again last night, fighting off the "baddies."
Often when I awake in the night, the evil one tries to crawl
in through my emotional chinks. All the words I usually say
seemed hollow and empty. I clung to the crucifix, repeating
over and over, "Lord Jesus Christ, Son of the living God,
have mercy on me, a sinner," and renouncing the temptations as they came: self-pity, fear, and the desire to control.

The final onslaught had to do with the fear that all these
changes in responsibilities and relationships are *only* the result of the effects of MS on my mind, not because they are
God's will for me. This is truly my hidden terror. When
the devil began attacking on this front, I sprang out of bed,
grabbed the holy water, and flung open the window and the
poustinia door to kick him out!

I finally managed to go back to sleep for a few hours.
When I awoke, I felt battered but victorious.

It was the victory of the cross. Aware, now, of the chinks,
which metamorphose into potholes on my spiritual path, I
know it is crucial to protect myself by constantly choosing
to trust and surrender. My heart has already said yes to this
call, but each time I seek satisfaction of emotional needs,
each time I play around with self-indulgence or choose a lesser good, I undermine the spiritual bulwark and open myself
to attack. The evil one tries to force his way into my mind,
but I can refuse him entrance.

Today my emotions are banged up, but it doesn't matter.
My body is a wreck—I was awakened by the aching in my
legs—but this doesn't matter either. Both body and emotions
are in Our Lady's hands.

July 26, 1999

I've no idea what has happened, but after almost two
weeks of pitched battle and intense inner pain, the struggle
has abated. Sushi has left for Hawaii to be with her mother,

who is dying. Last weekend, I found myself on and off with Janet and Katia. Their freshness and love were like balm on my heart.

God's grace is at work in my struggle, enabling the "yes" to be wrenched forth again and again. His grace is at work in people and circumstances. I need only to stand in the present moment and to let him act.

———•·•·•———

Madonna House Magadan Newsletter
from Janet Bourdet

August 5, 1999

Zdrastvuitye! Hello, Family!

For two weeks I couldn't even say hello to anyone here— the word was too hard to pronounce! But now, after seven weeks in Magadan, it's not the pronunciation that makes it so difficult to say good-bye. And since my return flight was cancelled and my departure postponed for another week, I'm going to pour myself a cup of tea and tell you a story about the Summer School of the Good Shepherd.

Two Sundays ago, I sat in church behind a weeping grandmother (*babushka* in Russian, with the accent on the first syllable). Why was she crying? I imagined something horrible. After the liturgy, she began talking with Marie, who motioned to me to come and listen. Marie translated as Babushka told us:

THE STORY OF A MUSTARD SEED

A pack of teenagers have been hanging out in the stair-well of her apartment. They spit on Babushka and call her names as she passes them. In her distress, she does some-thing most astonishing—she invites them to our little sum-mer school! They will be given lunch, she tells them, and offers to pay their bus fare.

A mustard seed has fallen out of Babushka's heart. Watered by her tears and their spittle, it begins to grow.

Week One

Bored and hungry, the stairwell gang arrives at the chapel.

"Who are these teenagers?" I ask. No one has ever seen them before. They look tough, underfed, and over-exposed to the very worst in life. I am afraid they will laugh me out of Russia when I bring out the miniature sheepfold, full of little sheep! They don't laugh, but towards the end of the week, someone confides to Kira, my teen-aged interpreter, that the stairwell gang is bored.

Kira is indignant. "How can they be bored? *I'm* not bored!"

The rest of the team decides a half-hour of games outside the chapel might enliven things a bit.

Week Two

During lunch a few of the stairwell gang sneak out for a cigarette. They are caught and told to leave because they have broken the rules. They ask forgiveness and literally beg to be allowed to stay.

The mustard seed is becoming a shrub.

Another day a fist fight breaks out during a game of tag. The girl says she is sorry, but the boy refuses her apology and runs off, crying. That's the last we'll see of Stas, I say to myself. He is far too cool to come back and face us after having been reduced to tears by a punch from a girl. But fifteen minutes later, there he is at the lesson, apologizing for his behaviour.

From the shelter of the mustard seed shrub, two birds are singing a new tune.

Middle of Week Two

A quiet peace descends on the room. Our meditations on the Good Samaritan and on the Publican and the Pharisee have been deep and sincere. The children have lots of questions: "What is mercy?" "How do you love those you hate you?" "Why can't we see God *now*?" "How good do you have to be to get into heaven?"

After the presentation of the Last Supper, I ask, "Why do we believe Jesus' words, 'This is My Body, this is My Blood'?"

Silence.

Then Simeon raises his hand. Kira leans over to translate his words into my ear, "'Because IT IS TRUE!'"

The mustard shrub grows three feet in that great and holy silence before a clamour of Russian voices bursts forth.

"What's going on?" I ask Kira. "What are they saying?"

"They are saying, 'THE LIGHT IS STRONGER THAN THE DARKNESS!'"

Week Three

No question about it; a mustard tree is standing big and branchy in the room. The kids ask if they can stay inside and work instead of playing outdoor games. Dasha, an eight-year-old prophetess, articulates what we are all feeling: "The joy of the mustard seed and the kingdom of heaven is so great, I HAVE TO GO SHARE IT WITH OTHERS!"

This was what had reduced Babushka to tears.

With love from Russia,
Janet, for Marie, Trudy, Miriam, Katia, and Sushi
(who is with her mother)

———

August 22, 1999

It is always difficult up at the *dacha*, where it is harder to walk and where my limitations are so exposed. I'm always grateful when we are "just us" or else with people who know me.

The feeling of vulnerability and humiliation at being so disfigured and dependent is overwhelming. All I can do is to fix my inner gaze on the disfigured Christ.

August 31, 1999

Yesterday I tripped and fell against the cement blocks by the garbage bins. I didn't really hurt myself, but it shook me up.

That evening Aquilina came and recounted once again her stories of miraculous survival in the camps. What struck me this time was her response to the camp authorities who were flailing about for explanations of why she hadn't frozen to death. "You say there is no God, but look—*God is! God is!*" she told them.

"This woman is going to get us all into heaven," Marie said later.

September 5, 1999

After a night of spasms, I read the line from Psalm 94, "Let us kneel before the God who made us." It came to me that I was created so that I might offer God this illness and all it entails, day by day, in atonement and intercession. This is my road to fulfillment: finding unity with Christ, intimacy in love, on the marriage bed of the cross.

I can truthfully say there is joy in this. Not emotionally, and usually not in the midst of pain, although once in a while, I do remember what it is all about. But on the spiritual level, there is an inner joy, for I have discovered the purpose of my life. *"I have given you the gift you asked for...."*

Maxim

In mid-September Marie, Trudy, Katia, and I attended the second pastoral conference for priests and religious in Irkutsk. Irkutsk was only four hours by plane from Magadan, but since we couldn't get a direct flight, we went by way of Krasnoyarsk, where we overnighted with the Claretian Fathers.

A young Russian seminarian named Maxim met us at the door of the Claretian residence. When we introduced ourselves as being from Madonna House, his mouth dropped open in astonishment and delight.

"Madonna House! I've been looking all over for you, and you have come to me!"

Maxim had come across the book *Poustinia* in East Germany, where his father was a political officer with the Soviet army. He subsequently read all of Catherine's books that he could find, both in Russian and in English. He loved Madonna House spirituality.

After breakfast the next morning, Maxim offered to take us to see an Orthodox chapel overlooking the city. The driver for the Claretians would take me in his car, and the others would go on foot.

"How did you hurt your leg?" Maxim wanted to know.

"I have multiple sclerosis."

He stared at me. Around us everyone was silent. Finally he put out his hand, palm upwards.

"You, too?" I asked incredulously.

He nodded.

There were tears in my eyes. There were tears in his eyes. In fact, there were tears in everyone's eyes.

"I am leading you."

A week after our return from Irkutsk, I came down with an intestinal infection that was making the rounds. Dr. Nelly thought it was salmonellosis. I found it particularly frightening when my fever exacerbated the MS symptoms for a couple days. I moved over to the main apartment. For a week, I lived on dried bread cubes, rice, and tea. Since I was getting pretty hungry, and since I was feeling better, Marie and Katia, both of whom were nurses, agreed I could have a hard-boiled egg. It tasted heavenly, but Nelly scolded us, saying that eggs were known to aggravate intestinal problems. Although the original infection had been cleared up with antibiotics, I now ended up with an acute intestinal inflammation. As the diarrhoea continued, I became so weak on the prescribed diet of more bread cubes, rice, and tea that, unbeknownst to me, I was on the verge of being hospitalized.

At first, I was too sick to do anything except give it all to God. Marie suggested I pray to Ksenia of St. Petersburg for healing, which I did. On October first, the feast of the Little Flower, I awoke without stomach pain for the first time and felt I'd turned a corner. Fr. Michael brought me communion and the sacrament of the sick. He also blessed the new apartment, which, to my surprise, was to be named in honour of St. Therese of the Child Jesus.

The whole day was a gift from St. Therese. I felt she had healed me, she and Ksenia...I hoped Ksenia didn't mind my giving so much credit to Therese! Then I pictured the two of them, arm in arm in heaven, laughing together at my concern. The communion of saints!

Fr. Michael brought the Blessed Sacrament into the bedroom while I rested. Lying in the warmth of God's gaze, I heard him say in my heart, *"Don't be afraid. I am leading you."*

October 18, 1999

Yesterday after Sunday Mass, I presented the new Russian edition of *Fragments of My Life* to the congregation. Although I knew what I wanted to say, I suddenly found myself wandering off. Was I just tired, or was it the effect of the MS? The fear that my brain is affected is greater than the fear of not being able to walk.

But if I can no longer speak as I used to, then the Lord is inviting me to be silent. I can offer this for Russia. I can offer everything. But I must stay "inside" it, eschewing self-observation and standing squarely before God in my heart. Perhaps this is why he is leading me to adoration.

October 25, 1999

I awoke during the night of Saturday to Sunday in such a state of anxiety that I couldn't even pray my usual prayer of offering. Suddenly I realized, *the offering has already been made.* It has been accepted. What I am experiencing is the reality of living it out. It's okay to be afraid....

Magadan Newsletter from Marie Javora

November 17, 1999

Dear Family,

It's been a long while since we've written, and I don't know how to begin to recap the past three months. At the time of writing, we are four— Miriam, Katia, Sushi, and I—but soon, we will once again be in transition. Next week Miriam leaves for Moscow on publication business and to renew apostolic contacts there before continuing on to Combermere for her annual medical check. Trudy will be returning from Combermere at the end of the month. In mid-January Sushi is scheduled to spend some time studying Russian in our house in Washington.

Winter is upon us, and the temperatures have dropped to minus twenty Celsius. Soon our *dacha* will have a new wood-and-coal stove, ready for winter use as a poustinia, though I'm not sure if anyone besides Trudy will feel hardy enough to venture out there!

Katia has begun to study Russian with a teacher from the university, who comes twice a week.

Much of our time these days is spent running. Running to the appropriate department to renew our visas every three months, running to the department that takes care of our apartment building to get the sewage leak in the cellar fixed, running to the Justice Department with all the documents needed to get re-registered as a religious organization, running to pay the rent, electricity, sewage and cold water, and heating and hot water.

But this is nothing compared to what our friends have to contend with. The Russians who are living well constitute a very small minority, while some of our professionally-employed friends are still unable to buy the basic necessities. We are continually awed by what people carry in such a hidden and courageous way, but as the strain takes its toll, we see depression and despair creeping into people's lives. For some, it has led to alcoholism and all the horrors accompanying this disease.

Fr. Michael recently visited a prison three hundred kilometres from Magadan, where the son of one of our parishioners is serving his term. Food rations there are close to those of the gulag days. Father is arranging for regular shipments of food staples to be sent through the parish branch of Caritas, an international humanitarian aid organization.

In response to the needs around us, we have initiated a day of adoration at the house each Thursday from ten in the morning until five-thirty in the afternoon, and we are gradually inviting a few others to join us. As Jean Fox told us when she was in Magadan two years ago, we need to become a holocaust of prayer, bringing to the Lord all the hopeless situations people bring to us.

At the parish, Fr. Michael is exposing the Blessed Sacrament on the Sundays of Advent from after Mass until 7 P.M., after which those present will be invited to a simple supper. The littlest and poorest are the ones most likely to be there praying to the end. What a beautiful way to prepare for the coming of our Saviour!

With love in Our Lady
and gratitude for our bond of love and unity,
Marie, for Sushi, Miriam, Katia, and soon—Trudy

COMBERMERE

Jesus Christ—today, yesterday, and forever

January 2, 2000

A century, a millennium has ended, and I am more incapable than ever of grasping the implications. To the relief of most, the fear of a world-wide computer glitch causing global havoc seems to have been a false alarm. I suppose no one can wish for catastrophe when you think of the real suffering it would bring, but I can't help but feel a little regret that the technological age wasn't shown to be fallible. We might have learned something.

At Midnight Mass we prayed for all the nations of the world, invoking God's mercy for the people of every country on this earth. How many Masses are being celebrated tonight across the globe, I wondered. How many Masses have been celebrated in all the centuries since Christ offered his Body and Blood for the life of the world?

For almost two thousand years, his mercy has been poured out upon this poor human race. Two thousand years of love, despite all the ways in which we have scorned his love and will continue to scorn it. We are sinners and will continue to sin, and still our Saviour goes in search of the lost sheep, of the heart that is hungry. This has little to do with our fidelity—and everything to do with his.

The meaning of the next millennium, or as long as it takes until the world ends, is God's love poured out on each human being, his offer of eternal life for the taking, love here and now for the taking. It is not a civilization that is redeemed, but each man and woman.

MAGADAN

Consoling the disfigured Christ

May 2, 2000

Several weeks ago, on Good Friday, we watched the end of the video *The Gospel according to St. Matthew*. I haven't been able to get it out of my mind. This is a human, masculine, tender Jesus, full of joy and deep, warm love. But as the Passion unrolls, all this disappears, and Jesus truly becomes "a man to make people screen their faces" (Is 53:3). It's the first time I have understood what he looked like in those hours that changed the course of human history.

It is this disfigured, bloodied Jesus, stripped of all his allurement and charisma, before whom I am called to stand, whom I am called to recognize in the bloodied, swollen faces of the alcoholics on the street, in the sick and the suffering. Do I choose to be there with him?

———

From Fr. Michael's homily at a Saturday morning Mass

We can't begin to fill the needs of these times. So what can we do? We can take the suffering, the anger, the divisiveness into ourselves, saying, "It stops here," and lift it up to God. This is what we are called to live.

Jesus didn't save the world by his miracles or healings, but by his death on the cross. It was when he was weakest that he saved us.

May 15, 2000

We are reeling from the rape, torture, and murder of Tanya Kononova's ten-year-old pupil Maria, who was also the classmate of several children in our parish. Her assailant had followed her home from school, somehow gaining access to the apartment. She was an only child and lived with her mother, who was at work when the tragedy took place.

All the gnawing dissatisfactions that distract me from the essentials have fallen away, stripped of their power. We are here for one purpose only: to carry the cross for and with these people.

As we returned from Tanya's on the night of the murder, God gave me an incredible grace. Into my mind came the image of Christ in the video, crucified and "so disfigured he seemed no longer human." Suddenly little Maria's body was his body—his disfigured body was Maria's. It didn't take away the pain, but it changed it.

At Mass on Sunday, Fr. Michael waited until the very end of the liturgy before referring to the event that was foremost in everyone's mind. Instead of the final blessing, he invited all those who wished to receive the sacrament of the sick to come forward. "Today all our hearts need healing," he said quietly.

No human words could have touched the pain. Only Christ, crucified and risen, can turn the brokenness to love. He alone can defeat evil.

The whole congregation surged forward. The choir sang the *Magnificat*, and as we went into the Taizé canon "Ave Maria," I went to get music for the "Song of Songs," not knowing that this was what Polina herself wanted to sing.

"Come then, my love, my lovely one come." Come, little Maria. You have truly washed your robe in the blood of the Lamb. The moment of your agony is past, and God will wipe away your tears while you drink forever at the spring of living water.

May 16, 2000

Trudy came over to the poustinia this morning to tell me there had been another murder. Same pattern, but this time it was a young woman. They think they have caught the perpetrator.

Later in the day we learned that our *dacha* and storage shed were broken into. Roofing materials, both sleeping bags, and a pillow were taken. Everything was thrown about; the prayer books were ruined.

To add to all the tragedies, Nadia's daughter lost the baby she was carrying.

May 22, 2000

Little Maria's funeral at the Orthodox church was attended by an enormous number of people. Many children came on their own, without an adult. Classes had been cancelled at Tanya's school, where the *paminki*, the memorial meal, was to be held after the burial. Tanya had organized everything. She told us that each time she goes into a store, people hand her money for Maria's mother. The municipal government will be giving the latter a new apartment.

With the funeral over and the slayer arrested, the emotion and fear in the city seem to have subsided. What remains is a sober reminder of the spiritual battle in which we live, and the intensified call to give ourselves completely.

June 14, 2000

I stopped by Nina's on the way home from Mass last night and ended up staying for supper. We were talking about Olga, who had been in the camps, and who had been telling us last week how she and other Lithuanian students in Lvov had been rounded up and charged with nationalist activities.

"What had she done?" Nina wanted to know.

"Why, nothing – she hadn't done anything!"

"But if she was convicted, she must have done something."

I couldn't believe what I was hearing. "She was totally innocent, Nina. So was Bronislava. None of them were guilty of anything."

I had been told that many people still think the political prisoners must have been guilty of wrongdoing, or else they would not have been in the camps. Still, it was shocking to hear it from someone so close to us, in reference to a fellow parishioner whom she knows and loves.

June 26, 2000

Katia and Trudy have returned from this year's retreat for women religious in Irkutsk and from Maxim's diaconal ordination in Krasnoyarsk. They are brimming over with new impressions and experiences. They were particularly struck by the interest in Madonna House among those whom they met.

The hard truth is that I am jealous. I long to be on the apostolic cutting edge again. I long to travel, to touch the life of this country in all its dimensions. I was beginning to do all this before the MS diagnosis; now I am blocked.

Last night I woke up crying and couldn't get back to sleep. The only truth I could grasp was my identification with those who had perished in Kolyma, in the other labour camps, and yes, in the Nazi concentration camps as well. This identification is my deep vocation, the meaning of my life. But it isn't what I would have chosen.

June 27, 2000

Last night I awoke with a sense of deep peace. Into my half-consciousness came the words, *"Why are you trying so hard? I am carrying you."*

Marie

In early July Trudy left on holidays and to spend a few months in Combermere.

Marie had remained in Combermere after the Directors' Meetings to make a forty-day Ignatian retreat. She had left Magadan in a state of exhaustion, and we had been hoping she would also get a good rest. Now that she was back, it wasn't clear whether or not the break had replenished her physically, but the peace emanating from her spirit embraced us all.

"When I pray about our house," she told us, "it comes to me that in Russia, Christian faith was strengthened, above all, through the lives of holy men and women. Here in Magadan, our spirituality is not going to be communicated verbally, but *through our inner dying and resurrection.* If we allow this to happen in us, the hope to which we are called to witness will shine in our very being."

Marie's gift of self was total, but by the middle of August, her fatigue was again so noticeable that Katia, Sushi and I were concerned. She who so rarely complained began speaking of a constant headache and dizziness. When she developed pharyngitis, we called Dr. Nelly, who noticed a slight droop in the corner of Marie's mouth. Nelly thought she had had a T.I.A., a warning sign of a possible impending stroke, and put Marie on strict bed rest.

We were stunned at the implications of Marie's condition. To think that she might have to leave Magadan was almost unbearable. Her heart was totally invested in our life, and her spiritual gifts, now in full fruition, were uniquely adapted to this apostolate and culture. But this was a time to stay centered in the moment, clinging to God and brushing aside the anxieties that buzzed like flies in our hearts.

Each of us stood with Marie in our own way. Katia, a nurse, was caring for her with great attentiveness and sensitivity. Between Marie and me, the spiritual bond had so deepened during the years we had been together that now we did not even need words.

It had been no accident that on the feast of the Assumption, I had had a sense of the Lord giving his Mother to me. We needed her especially now. She had shared Christ's suffering; she was the Queen of Compassion. In her, we were one with each other, one in compassion.

August 22, 2000, feast of the Queenship of Mary

I guessed, even before she told me, that Marie is leaving. She herself is still trying to digest the reality.

For all of us, grief is just beneath the surface. I went to the church office to ask Lyuba for an official letter requesting an emergency exit visa for Marie. When I saw the tears in Lyuba's eyes, I almost broke down myself.

Nelly is trying to determine to what extent, if any, Marie's symptoms are a reaction to the Magadan climate. I don't know which would be worse – a pre-stroke condition necessitating months of rest, after which she *might* be able to come back, or a climate-related condition precluding any return to Magadan.

I can't imagine the next months without her.

In an e-mail yesterday, Jean reflected that in the event that no one can withstand the climatic pressures here, we might have to close the house and reopen a centre elsewhere in Russia. The thought strikes terror in my heart. How could we abandon these people, this parish?

To run the house, we need at least two able-bodied people with a call to poustinia, at least one of them able to learn Russian, and both with the desire to give their lives totally. As Marie observed dryly, there don't seem to be many candidates.

Yesterday Marie put Katia in charge until they leave for Canada. I understand the reasons, but it is more salt in my wound.

Lord, I offer you my humiliation, my inadequacy. Help me to stay out of my head; help me to stand in my heart, in the pain, and to give it to you for Marie, for our house, for Magadan.

Jean had written that Trudy would be staying in Combermere for an extended period of time.. Marie herself would be away for at least three to six months. Katia was flying with her to Combermere, and Jean felt strongly that full-time language study was Katia's next priority. This left Sushi and me in Magadan, and while Sushi had considerable natural energy, I could hardly move, even with ten hours of sleep each night and a rest each day.

The days pending Marie and Katia's departure were so heavy, so draining with the stream of good-bye visits, that we all longed for them to be over. Exhaustion was a merciful anaesthetic, dulling the drama and muffling emotions that would otherwise have been too overwhelming.

On September sixth Sushi left with the parish delegation to attend the consecration of the new cathedral in Irkutsk. Several hours later, Marie and Katia departed for the airport, en route to Anchorage and Combermere. Numb with the events of the past weeks, I was glad to be alone for a few days.

If Today You Hear His Voice (Ps. 94)

SEPTEMBER 2000

From a report by Sushi Horwitz

I was privileged to be in Irkutsk, the seat of our diocese, for the consecration of the new Cathedral of the Immaculate Heart of Mary.

At the heart of the three-day celebration were the "Confessors" of the gulag. Each day the spiritual intensity increased. On Saturday afternoon the recitation of the rosary was interspersed with witnesses from elderly camp survivors, including our own Bronislava and Olga, of how Our Lady had helped them during their years of suffering. One of the older parishioners in our Magadan contingent said she had never before realized the truth of what had transpired in her country.

Sunday Mass was offered by eighty-seven-year-old Cardinal Kasimir Swiatek, archbishop of Minsk in Belarus, who spent fifteen years in prison and in the camps, including a stint on death row. This was his first visit to Siberia as a free man.

Archbishop Kondrusiewicz from Moscow preached the homily and wept as he shared the experience of seeing the cathedral in his native city razed. He called us each to help restore the faith and the Church in Russia. At the end of his homily, he went over and embraced the cardinal, saying, "He too shared in the suffering." This brought the cardinal to tears, and they held each other for a long time.

After Mass, Cardinal Swiatek led the procession from the cathedral to the outdoor Chapel of Peace and Reconciliation, dedicated to those who had suffered and died in the camps. The memorial consists of fourteen stone markers representing the Stations of the Cross. Each marker bears the name of a camp and beneath it is an urn. One of these markers reads "Magadan-Kolyma."

When the cornerstone for the cathedral was blessed last year, handfuls of earth were brought from various labour camps in the diocese, including from around the ice cells outside Magadan. Now, with his bare hands, the aged cardinal carefully scooped the earth from each of fourteen bowls into the corresponding urn. The urn was covered, and the cardinal lit a vigil lamp by each marker. After lighting the lamp next to the name of the camp where he himself had been interned, he covered his face with his hands, and his body shook with silent sobs. Our Bishop Jerzy helped him back to the microphone. When he had finished the official prayers, the cardinal leaned his head against his staff and stood bowed with grief...

———

On September fourteenth, the feast of the Exaltation of the Cross, and the seventh anniversary of Madonna House in Magadan, more members of the team were in Combermere than here in Russia. No one but God could have arranged this scenario.

The following day, Sushi and I received an e-mail from Jean:

Neither of you will be in charge. Instead, see this as a time to bow before one another, love one another, and communicate as peers for the good of the house and of all who come. Live in harmony, give way to each other, and many graces will follow. Trust in God's mercy as never before, and stay very faithful to the cross. Surrender everything into the heart of Our Lady. She is at work.

Neither of you will be in charge. This was the last thing either of us had expected, but it was an inspired decision, relieving both of us of our authority problems. Jean also told us that when I left in December for my winter rest and medical appointments in Canada, Alma would come to be with Sushi.

In confession a few weeks previously, Fr. Michael had told me, "Each time you are tempted to want authority, remember the rich young man. He was afraid to sell all he possessed, and he went away with nothing."

It had always been the challenge of responsibility that attracted me, not the exercise of power. Now God was offering me a different challenge. He was asking me to renounce the security of a role so that he might give me the security of living in the Spirit.

From a letter to Jean, October 30, 2000

...The house has been quiet. Some days there are no visitors at all, and even our Wednesday rosary gatherings seem quieter. Nevertheless, Alma's arrival will be timely. Although Sushi and I have been doing well together—much better than we or anyone expected—it isn't a normal community life by a long shot.

We are out of the humanitarian aid apostolate almost completely. We still give some food each month to our Old Believer friends, Matushka and her son Nikola, and we help with his medicines. I am continuing our practice of sending periodic parcels to our prisoner friend, Alek Turkin, who is serving a twelve-year sentence in a prison near the airport. Both Nikola and Alek can be like thorns in our sides, but they help us to remember that we, too, have been given everything.

Fr. Michael is hoping to start construction of the church in the spring. Much as people like the intimacy of our little chapel, it is important to them that we have a real church building.

On the feast of the Rosary, when Sushi and I renewed our consecration to Our Lady at the end of Saturday evening adoration at the parish, I found myself entrusting our apostolate and all that we are living into the hands of the Mother of God. So often it feels as if our personal limitations constrict our ability to do much more than simply live. However, it seems to me, more and more, that simply living *is* our vocation in Magadan.

"You are all different, but you all love," Nina said yesterday. And another friend told us, "Just to know you're here, that I can come when I need to, and that you pray for me—this means everything."

Nadia was halfway out the door after the Wednesday night rosary when she turned and said, "You give us so much. You give us peace and hope. I sometimes wonder, what do we leave with you when we go?"

Sushi just about choked. "If you have a few hours, I'll tell you!"

Yesterday at the parish, I overheard a woman who was not even especially close to us say, "Madonna House is an example for me that a single woman can live chastely in the world, with honesty and dignity." This is the first time I've ever heard anyone in Magadan reflect on our charism as laywomen.

We did not come here to change people, but to love them. It is immaterial whether or not we speak the language well, or whether there are five of us or only two. Our apostolic work is to love each other and each person we meet, to receive God's love in all the ways it comes, and to pass it on through our presence, our self-giving, our way of life, and our prayer. It is this, not anything we do, that matters.

COMBERMERE

When I arrived in Combermere in December, what a joy to be reunited with Marie! But awaiting me was yet another challenge. Jean had given Trudy and Katia permission to travel in western Russia and the Baltic countries, where they would "sniff the Spirit," as Jean put it. They would be continuing, in a sense, the apostolic outreach I had begun in Moscow and Latvia, but which, clearly, was no longer God's will for me. That I had not completely accepted this was evidenced by my jealousy.

Your will for me now is the cross. Only by uniting myself with your will can I remain united with my sisters.

January 8, 2001

This poustinia day has been a struggle. The weight of the cross is heavy, and I've lost my bearings. I can't force my feelings, but with my will, I embrace the cross.

We've come too far, Lord. There's no turning back.

Jesus says, *"I'm part of you now. Your cross is my cross. My cross is your cross. Put your hand in mine. We will carry it together."*

February 5, 2001

Last night I had painful upper leg spasms, the worst yet, leaving me weak, tired, teary, and dependent on the Lord. I tried to offer it for Trudy and Katia.

Thank you, Lord, for the past two months of relative well-being, sound sleep, and increased energy. This has been your gift, and I will try not to hang on to it. Physical pain such as I experienced last night unites me with you more directly than anything else.

February 27, 2001 – Shrove Tuesday

Several weeks ago the "Combermere Magadaners"– Marie, Trudy, Katia, and I–met with Jean to discuss the Russian apostolate and Trudy and Katia's mission. A new movement of the Spirit is beginning with them; we will see where God leads and what he opens for the future of Madonna House in Russia.

Back in Magadan, a new phase is beginning. Fr. Michael will be increasingly involved with the construction of the new church and probably less available to us. We must listen carefully to hear what God is asking of us.

When Jean invited each of us to share what was in her heart, I spoke of my pain in abandoning an active apostolic role. But yesterday, at the farewell Mass for Katia and Trudy, cutting through everything else in my heart came the words, *"This venture is God's work, contingent on nothing else."*

It isn't a matter of "if I didn't have MS" or "if things had happened differently." This is God's plan, and not only must I accept it, I must unite myself to it and rejoice in it. Otherwise I am not in God's will.

They have been chosen for this next step, just as Marie, Alma, and I were chosen for the first step. God is asking me to bless this venture from the heart of my own freedom.

March 5, 2001

Yesterday I awoke with the ringing of the alarm after another night of severe spasms. All day I felt as if I'd been beaten up.

There is something terrifying about these solitary, hidden, nights of pain. Terrifying and intimate. Last night I prayed Sunday compline which includes Psalm 90, *"He who dwells in the shadow of the Almighty,"* and I knew God would not allow my foot to slip. The night, though still not restful, was better. *"For I will set my angels around you, to guard you in all your ways."*

March 19, 2001

Another mild, sunny spring day. Everyone here is taking advantage of the beautiful weather to go for walks. I went walking a bit (which isn't very much), then simply stood in the parking lot, leaning on my cane. This made me think of our grannies in Magadan, who do exactly the same thing. I longed to be back in Russia.

I suppose lack of awareness is better than pity, but once in a while, it would be consoling if someone were to ask, "Is it hard for you not to be able to enjoy the fresh air?" Of course, this isn't done; one waits for the handicapped person to bring it up, and I never do, because most people wouldn't know how to react.

It is important not to have expectations. This is the cross and it won't go away. Only I can carry it—with Christ. And just now, the pain is too great to dwell upon.

"No one takes [my life] from me. I lay it down of my own free will." (Jn 10:17-18)

I did not do this well today.

I do offer it, Lord, in union with you, for all those whose lives are truncated by circumstances or history; for all those who cannot go where their own desires, talents, and potential would naturally lead them.

MAGADAN

May 14, 2001

I am finally back. Magadan has never seemed so grey.

Fr. Michael came to supper on Thursday and talked about the conflicts and personal crises in our parish community. He talked and talked. Finally, lacing up his boots to go, he said, "If, every morning when I wake up, I say to God, 'I am yours,' and keep returning to this throughout the day, then I know that the battle is his and not mine. God knows what is happening, and he is working in the midst of it. I can let him use me."

This is true for us all.

It seems to me that in this house, we are all victim souls. Sushi, Alma, and I are all handicapped in different ways—physically, emotionally, linguistically—and none of us are living according to our human talents and desires. We can offer this in love and compassion for the people of Magadan. Few of them are doing what they would choose to do, were circumstances different.

May 18, 2001

Today I heard in my heart, *"If today you hear his voice, open your heart to be taught by the Spirit."* This is really where we all have to stand. We can try to accept each other's weaknesses, but the greater challenge is to listen for the Holy Spirit speaking through each other.

May 28, 2001

Fr. Michael was telling us today that each time he thinks he has the parish organized and the right people in place, it all falls through. Someone in a key position has a drinking spree, a catechist drops out without warning or explanation, etc., etc. In the end, however, these situations are bringing Fr. Michael closer to the people. He is finding that he is just as broken as anyone else.

The difference is that they have a basic trust we lack. How often have we heard our friends say, "Never mind—

we'll manage. We'll get through this." Not understanding the underlying heroism of their lives, they continue to get up early day after day, pouring themselves out and, unbeknownst to themselves, living the Gospel.

We identify with them by getting up each morning with MS or a language handicap or the sense of not being able to do the kind of work we would wish. We can't escape our limitations any more than our Russian friends can escape theirs. We draw strength from them and from our community life.

June 27, 2001

Toli has been released early from prison, and last night, after Mass, we celebrated his twenty-seventh birthday and the beginning of his new life. Instead of having been destroyed by his two years in the penal camp, as we had all feared—and not without reason—he has emerged with new strength. What a witness to the power of prayer and God's fidelity.

August 6, 2001, Feast of the Transfiguration

Two days ago we received the following e-mail from Marie in Combermere:

> Jean just walked through the office and asked me to tell you that she is appointing Beth Holmes as director in Magadan. This seems a real inspiration on Jean's part, and I trust it entirely. She believes it will help stabilize the house at this time.

Beth, otherwise known as Liza, fell in love with Russia in 1995, when she came to Magadan to help us out. She will have to learn the language and everything else as well, but we can all work together and help each other.

What I have just written is the mature reaction I struggle to maintain. Emotionally, it cuts like a sword, a bitter reminder that I am no longer able to carry the apostolate I knew better than any of us.

Lord, help me to stay in the truth. Help me to renounce, once and for all, my pretensions to leadership. This is not where you are calling me.

On the afternoon of September twelfth, I was in the publications office, trying to make sense of an e-mail that had just come in from Combermere, in which Jean made a reference to an attack a few hours previously on the Twin Towers in New York City. I calculated the time difference: 9 A.M. on September eleventh in New York would have been one o'clock this morning in Magadan. I was still trying to figure out what she was talking about when Liza came in, her face ashen.

"Fr. David just phoned," she said. "There have been terrorist attacks in the U.S. Two planes rammed into the Twin Towers in New York and another into the Pentagon in Washington, D.C. A fourth plane was also on its way to Washington, but seems to have crashed in Pennsylvania."

We stared at each other in disbelief. I showed her the letter from Jean. Suddenly remembering that there was a 1 P.M. newscast, we raced to the other apartment and switched on the TV just in time to see the horrendous replays of the two towers slowly imploding.

Compassion for those who suffer was one of the most beautiful of all Russian traits, and throughout the day people kept phoning us to express their condolences and solidarity. At the same time, we sensed that a reflex of fear had been activated. People prayed at Mass that there would not be a third world war. They feared America's power, and they knew what war meant.

October 29, 2001

It is dizzying to keep up with all the changes. To our joy and the joy of our friends, Marie is back in Magadan. With Liza as Local Director, supported by Marie's wisdom and experience, the house is in a much healthier position.

After travels in Latvia and Ukraine, during which she and Trudy made many contacts and acquired valuable experience, Katia is staying on in Moscow to study Russian. She will need a solid foundation in the language for whatever the future holds, and there is really no way for her to study while actively involved in apostolic work.

Trudy's migraines have become so debilitating that she has had to return to Combermere for treatment. Alma is also back in Combermere.

Marie keeps reminding me that my present life is the spiritual underpinning of the house. "It's not just your publishing work that is important," she reiterates.

I need to accept my limitations, not as a personal loss but as something to be offered *willingly*, through the power of the Spirit, for the house and the world. In this knowledge lies the freedom and joy with which I so want to live.

God doesn't want suffering, but transforms it. He gathers up the fragments of our fallen life so that nothing we experience can separate us from him. Although I cannot say with undivided conviction, "I prefer death in Christ Jesus to anything the world has to offer," I desire to be able to say this, and I believe Christ is helping me.

COMBERMERE

A *"prisoner"* for the Lord
December 27, 2001

Yesterday I was working at my desk when Jean Fox appeared in the doorway.

"I've just had an e-mail from Magadan," she said. "Marie and Beth want to reduce the house activity for six months so that they can concentrate on studying Russian. Beth *has* to learn," she added.

"What does that mean—'reduce the house activity?'"

"They want to try to simplify life as much as possible. Trudy won't be going back. Her health won't allow it. Alma is staying here in any case. Sushi will be coming for a couple months. And they want you to stay until after the Directors' Meetings in May."

"Stay in Combermere until after May?" I tried to keep my voice steady, but my world was coming apart. Magadan *was* my world; I belonged there. How could they cast me out?

What Jean wasn't saying, what didn't have to be said because it was so obvious, was that if they were trying to pare down everything in order to have time to study, my presence would be a burden. With just the two of them, as long as there wasn't a lot of outside activity, they could manage. But I couldn't cook or clean or do my own laundry. I would need help.

Last fall Marie had spoken to me about the necessary compromises, when a person is sick or handicapped, between the person's own needs and the long-term needs of the apostolate. Was this one of those instances? Then what about all she had said about my suffering being the backbone of the house?

Now I understood why my phone conversation with Marie a few days before had been so lacking in clarity. Why hadn't she just said, "Things are happening here, but I can't explain until we hear from Jean?" Was I not part of the house? If it had been explained to me, I would not have opposed it.

"Can you offer this as a sacrifice for the house is Magadan, for the future of Madonna House in Russia?" Jean asked softly.

I nodded. I couldn't trust myself to talk.

The sense of betrayal and rejection is devastating.

December 29, 2001

I don't know any of the details, and I am afraid of the anger and resentment that are clamouring for entry into my heart. The greatest temptation is towards division.

Two years ago, Marie told me, "Because we are one, you are part of what we are living. Unity transcends time and space. It is not geographical." I am one with Liza and Marie to the extent that I can accept this decision as God's will for me.

I know what he is asking, but my understanding is crucified, not to mention my emotions. It has to be an act of
faith.

December 31, 2001
The last day of the year. I am still locked in my inner
battle, but at least it is the struggle to stay before God, to
surrender to *him*, to keep the battle on the front where it
belongs.

Early mornings, as I lie in bed, are the worst. I can't
think my way out of the pain.

January 3, 2002
*"Pray for us, too, that God may provide us with an opening to
proclaim the mystery of Christ, for which I am a prisoner. Pray that I
may speak it clearly, as I must."* (Col. 4:3-4)

I too feel like a prisoner for Christ. Alma says I am "under house arrest."

I am in exile, my home ripped away from me.

*Lord, did you have to let those words surface, reminding me that
this is my spiritual tie with those in the camps?*

January 4, 2002
God knows the depth of my love for Magadan and my
desire to be there. Is he not purifying this passionate desire
so that my relationship with him might be first?

A few days ago at Mass, the words came to me, *"What
you are living will bear fruit."* It is the cross, and the cross saved
the world.

To stay on the cutting edge of the pain and to keep offering it without falling into self-pity requires vigilance. I
need to repent of my anger. God is calling me to live in his
kingdom.

January 7, 2002
Last night I dreamt of a bird whose brain was too lim-
ited to take the weight of having to translate the songs of St.
Therese of Lisieux and who died "in anxiety and despair!"

This "birdbrain" is me. God is pointing to a way that cannot be grasped by my human intellect, and if I persist in trying to do so, I should not be surprised at the consequences. Anxiety and despair are definitely two of the spirits tempting me.

January 11, 2002

I'm not sure what has happened; but I think I have crossed a Rubicon. I feel a steadiness that wasn't there before, an inner stillness and peace, as if I am moving on a wave of grace.

God asks me to live this moment only—with him, for him and through him.

From a letter to Marie, January 15, 2002

I've just finished a private retreat, using Catherine's writings. I never expected it to affect me so powerfully. The readings seemed to address my present struggle. Although I had assented to the request that I stay in Combermere for the coming months, the emotional pain has been tearing me apart. There was a step I couldn't take—and perhaps didn't want to take.

On the very first day of the retreat, I found myself sobbing and sobbing. If Catherine's surrender was so vital for the salvation of priests, then I can't pretend that what God is asking of me is without consequence, albeit on a much lesser scale.

I have to acknowledge that God can accomplish what he wishes in Magadan, using whatever means he desires. He doesn't need me to be there. *He* is the Saviour. Since he is asking me to stay in Combermere for the good of our apostolate in Russia, it is crucial that I say yes.

No settling down

During Holy Week 2002, Marie began having symptoms similar to those she had suffered in 2000. The condition was later diagnosed as neutropenia, a disease in which there is an abnormally low number of a certain type of white blood cell. She managed to get through the week, and on Easter Tuesday, she and Liza left together for Moscow. They stayed with Katia for the next two days while Marie received massive intravenous doses of antibiotics at the American Clinic. Then Marie flew to Toronto, accompanied by Katia, and was admitted directly to hospital.

By the time they arrived in Combermere, two weeks later, Marie looked much better than I'd expected. She was, understandably, shaken by all that has happened.

Ours were not the only precarious destinies. Towards the end of April, Bishop Mazur was expelled from Russia, his year-long visa revoked without explanation at the Moscow airport as he was coming back from a visit to his native Poland. He had no choice but to take the return flight to Warsaw.

In Magadan the new Orthodox bishop appeared on TV and spoke of the sexual abuse scandals in the American Catholic Church. He said many priests had left their dioceses to avoid being brought to justice and implied that this might have been Fr. Michael's purpose in coming to Magadan.

I felt sick for Fr. Michael. *Lord, help me to offer everything.*

June 7, 2002

In two days, Liza will leave to begin a year of Russian studies in Washington D.C. Katia will be returning to Moscow to continue her own language studies, and Jean wants me to wait here in Combermere until Marie gets clearance from her doctor, hopefully at the beginning of July. Sushi, meanwhile, will be on her own in Magadan, staying with friends and also working on Russian. She is thrilled at the prospect.

I did not want to learn what this year has taught me—that even if my own health remains stable, *I can never again take it for granted that I can be in Magadan.*

Our lives are contingent on God's will. We can take nothing for granted. We can never settle down. This is what I have always found so hard to accept.

July 12, 2002

Marie and I met with Jean to talk about the return to Magadan.

Sushi will be the Local Director. Marie and I are called to pray for her and uphold her.

"Do not look for results from your work there," Jean told us, "If your lives are given to God, the people you are serving will receive light from you. Do not be afraid of suffering, weakness, or anything that might happen to you from without. In Magadan, the only joy is the joy of the cross. Bow low before each other."

I spoke with Marie later about the difficulty of living with a handicap in a community setting.

"It's humiliating," she agreed. And then, in a lowered tone, almost with a catch in her voice, she added, "And it's a very precious gift."

The gift of the Crucified. Will I accept it?

Little, Be Always Little

August 27, 2002

Dear Jean,

On every level we are being plunged deeper and deeper into the mystery that is Russia.

Almost nine years ago we arrived in Magadan without plans and without knowing what our apostolate would be. For the first few years, it was as if God were training us. Through the people, he showed us how to love without counting the cost. We sought to go the extra mile without hesitation, and we tasted the heady joy of trying to live the Gospel without compromise, even though we were eaten up and stretched beyond our physical and emotional limits.

When you visited us in December 1996, you saw that we were being swallowed up by our efforts to give material aid, and that this was not what God was calling us to. You told us that many people could do these works, but not everyone could become a holocaust.

The Western instinct is always to define needs and build accordingly. But Russia is not a very propitious place for builders. Century after century, everything gets swept away in a tide of destruction. Generation after generation has lived in the mystery of the cross.

God has granted our little apostolate the immense privilege of participating in this mystery. He has been making us small and poor so that he might use us. He is honouring our desire to give ourselves at the deepest level, and he offers us the possibility of identifying, in the depths of our being, with the redemptive suffering that seems to be Russia's call.

One of the great lessons to be learned from Russian spirituality is that of humility. Without humility, we cannot serve God. Perhaps we Catholics, who have not experienced the trials undergone by the Russian Orthodox Church in the last century, need to let our own hearts be purified—even by such apparent injustices as the recent expulsion of Bishop Jerzy.

It does look as if Fr. Michael will be allowed to remain in Magadan. Russia may be a land of suffering, but it is also a land of miracles!

People's joy at our return is ample evidence that all they want is for us to be here. They could care less about what we do. The very challenge of *being here* keeps us dependent on God.

Sushi has been praying to find people who can help with the cooking, laundry, and cleaning—friends who can fit into our daily life. Once I would have been mortified at the idea of paying someone to work for us. Now my understanding of identification is deeper—our overriding priority is to *be here*. It isn't what *we* do, but what *God* does, and we see him working through what might at first glance seem an uncomfortable situation.

Our first helper was Ira, an eighteen-year-old filled with life and faith, a member of Sushi's young people's group. When Ira had to quit in order to begin her university studies, Valya, a German-Russian in her fifties, agreed to help us, appreciative of the extra income. She grew up in Kazakhstan and came to Magadan with her husband five years ago. We now have become "her own," as the Russians say.

One day Valya brought her family photographs, including pictures of the maternal grandparents and aunts who starved to death in the 1931 famine precipitated by Stalin's mass collectivization plan. Another day she made *oladis*, a type of Russian pancake, and gathered us for an impromptu tea after morning adoration. Mindful of my weight, I declined a second helping. Valya, who is quite overweight herself, then quoted her mother as saying, "As long as there is food on the table—eat!" I thought of her grandparents and took the extra pancake.

Construction continues on our parish church. It will be beautiful! We are praying that it be ready for Christmas. As the government still won't let Bishop Mazur back into the country, he has asked that we postpone the consecration and just have a simple blessing for now.

Crazy as the house situation is, insecure as the ecclesial picture seems, I am more at peace than I have ever been. I deeply believe in the mystery we are living. It gives meaning and direction to my own life. To be here is an inestimable privilege, and I am grateful beyond words.

With my love and prayers,
Miriam

August 19, 2002

The three of us need to support each other, but not attempt to change or control each other. We cannot live in fear of each other's illnesses and neither should we feel responsible for them. This is what Jean meant when she urged us to stand together in our poverty. This is "littleness."

September 23, 2002

Last night at the rosary, I said something to Kostya about forgiving one of the parishioners, and he told me about seeing his mother decapitated with an electric wire when he was three years old. His father was in the next room, drunk. Kostya went on to describe the horrors of growing up in a state orphanage and ended, "This is why I can't forgive or pray for those who hurt me."

It was another reminder that I don't know what people are carrying, and I don't know what such experiences do to a person. I can only love and pray with all my being that the Father might pour his own healing love into the bruised and wounded heart of this young man.

November 11, 2002

Marie's health is sliding again. After the sauerkraut bee three weeks ago, she began to experience headache and dizziness. These have cleared up, but she almost fainted in chapel Sunday night and has continued to feel light-headed and generally unwell. She has been in touch with Combermere and with the doctor in Moscow who cared for her so skillfully last year. The whole scenario is charged with traumatic memories of her two previous crises.

We could hardly believe this was happening for the third time.

Throughout this incredibly intense and painful week, I marvelled as I watched Sushi move with the situation, one step at a time. Regardless of how helpless she must have felt before Marie's suffering, how unsure of what was needed, there were no outward signs of anxiety.

One day, as we gathered around Marie in chapel, Sushi began praying for her with an authority that surprised even her. Then, in the middle of a charismatic-style invocation, she suddenly broke off, saying, "This seems kind of weak—let's find a *real* prayer!" We all burst our laughing, but after that we began praying prayers of protection each day. We prayed for Marie's healing and peace and anointed her with the oil of Blessed Ksenia. Despite our growing concern, there was a unity and trust among the three of us that had never been there before.

Marie's physical and emotional distress was too acute for her to travel alone. Sushi phoned Katia in Moscow to bring her up to date on what was happening. Without being asked, Katia offered to fly to Magadan and accompany Marie back to Moscow for treatment at the American Clinic. Arriving the next day, Katia moved into the situation with grace and self-giving, bringing to it her own quality of lightness.

The next evening, as we finished praying the *Paraclesis,*˙ Marie asked us to remain in chapel, saying, "There is something I want to share with you." She told us that while walking alone earlier that afternoon, she had felt the grace of God breaking through the darkness that held her in its grip. She had heard in her heart the words, "Unless I go, the Holy Spirit cannot come to you." She now confirmed Sushi in her leadership, passing on the torch and adding that if she returned again, she felt it would only be for short periods of time.

---

* Byzantine-rite prayer service asking the intercession of the Mother of God for those who are suffering.

The power and clarity of that moment were indescribable. Although we were all choking back sobs, I saw the visible working of grace, of Marie's listening to the Spirit and responding with breathtaking totality. I saw the fruits of her faithfulness and of God's faithfulness to her and to all of us.

Although I had experienced many powerful spiritual moments, I had never experienced darkness turning so dramatically to light through a heart as pierced as Marie's. Her spiritual strength overshadowed the weakness of her body, transforming what, moments before, had seemed high tragedy into vision, clarity, and a shimmering sense of hope.

We were all stunned. And we too felt changed. It was as if Marie had taken the ray of light God had flashed into her heart and turned it into a stream of grace for us all.

One more phase of our Magadan apostolate had come to an end, and another was beginning. None of us had ever anticipated it happening this way. I had never thought that of the founding three, Marie would be taken and I would be left. I had even told God I was ready to sacrifice being in Magadan for Marie's sake. But he hadn't asked for that.

November 25, 2002

The terrible emptiness of the week after Marie's departure was broken by the sound of her voice on the telephone Monday night. Now Sushi and I are trying to steer a straight course before God and not swing back and forth emotionally with each new phone call.

Nor can we second guess the future. Jean has written that she has no one else to send to Magadan. We will have to live day by day, trusting in God. We can't stand before each other; we have to stand together before him.

Jean wrote to me in an e-mail:

The fact that you and Sushi are receiving graces is clearly a fruit of Marie's crucifixion. Marie has been a lightning rod for the Magadan apostolate. If she leaves Russia, someone else will have to assume that position. Who is ready for such suffering? We look at everything from a human perspective, but heaven is asking us to acquire new eyes, new ears, and a new heart.

Her words came as a challenge. I had a flashback to Edith Stein asking herself the question, "Who will atone for the Nazis? *I will!*" She died in a gas chamber the day she arrived in Auschwitz.

I wrote Jean that while I was far from having Marie's gifts, I offered myself completely for the Russian apostolate. Even the smallest of us could give our lives as a sacrifice.

The exchange of letters shook me to the core of my being.

December 2, 2002

After our Saturday morning Mass and tea, Bronislava and Olga, both of whom can hardly walk, were getting ready to attend a gathering of the camp survivors at the library. For the healthy, the library is only a five-minute walk from our apartment; for the lame, it takes a little longer. Thinking I was tired, Sushi suggested I go in a taxi—the ladies wouldn't be caught dead doing so! She reminded me that when I stretch myself too far, there are consequences for the house.

It was the kind of situation I find particularly painful: the need to determine my own limits and overcome my fears versus the call to sacrifice my independence for the good of the whole.

I chose to walk. It was good to listen to God while moving physically, a luxury I'm rarely able to enjoy now.

As I struggled with the strong emotions aroused by the incident, the thought kept surfacing: *acceptance of humiliation.* With it came an image of the humiliated Christ, who *"though he was God…did not deem equality with God something to be grasped at, but emptied himself to assume the condition of a slave…and being as all men are, he became humbler yet, even to accepting death, death on a cross."* (Phil 2:6-8)

It was a taste of intimacy, more precious than independence, more precious than anything in the world. I was on my way to a gathering of gulag survivors. Could anything have been more appropriate?

The Church of the Nativity of Christ

Since the Russian government was still adamant in its refusal to grant Bishop Mazur a visa, Fr. Michael had asked Archbishop Francis Hurley, recently retired from the see of Anchorage, to bless the new church when it opened before Christmas.

Sushi and I had been dreading the prospect of spending the holidays without reinforcements. The celebrations surrounding the opening, the visit of the archbishop, whom we knew so well, and the prospect of friends returning for the event from other parts of Russia all seemed much more than two people could handle. But despite our trepidation, we were carried by grace. It turned out to be one of the most joyful Christmases either of us had experienced.

The solemn move to the new church took place on the Sunday before Christmas. It was followed by a week of festive liturgies, a concert by the municipal *a capella* chorus, a gathering at the church with camp survivors, and a program to thank those who had participated in the construction. What a season of joy!

The beauty of the church took me by surprise. Width and height provided a sense of space. Light flooded the interior from two sets of windows flanking the altar on both sides and reaching almost to the ceiling, and from a row of round windows above the balcony. The whole sanctuary, including the altar, was of shining white marble. Filling the space above the gold-plated tabernacle, a large icon of the Nativity of Christ, filled with angels and painted in warm tones of red, green, orange, and gold, radiated the joy of Christ's birth. Higher still, reaching almost to the ceiling, hung an enormous replica of St. Francis's cross from San Damiano.

Joy and beauty, two qualities significantly lacking in Magadan and in people's lives—what greater gift could the Church offer her children?

I heard no regret at losing the intimacy of the old chapel. In this land so closely identified with Orthodoxy, for Catholics to have a real church was a sign of legitimacy. Its beauty was a source of pride. Polina's exclamation summed it up: "I wish I could live here all the time!"

February 3, 2003

There are no words to express what it has been like for me to stand by Fr. Michael in his present struggle.

In years past my soul caught fire from the passionate love burning in this priest, and the spark became in me a small flame—small, but steady. He fed me spiritually, guided me, and set me on course to offer my MS to God. Later, with the church construction consuming his energies, he became less present to us, but by then I no longer needed to lean on him either spiritually or emotionally. He gave me a vision of life with God—the same kind of vision Catherine had had. God took this and forged it in the fire of my disease, and the vision has become my own.

God is stripping Fr. Michael now, leading him into this spiritual desert that he might be drawn anew to the one he loves. I understand this because of what I have been given in Madonna House and because my own soul has been given life through Fr. Michael. It is as if I am being called to return to him what God has given me through him. The awesomeness of it brings me to my knees.

Our beautiful church looms before Fr. Michael as a money-consuming monster. He is tormented by the thought that it might have been built on a more modest scale. Is this true? Perhaps some things might have been done differently, but it seems to me that the obstacles to this church being built at all were so great that they would never have been overcome, had it not been God's will.

I know you are working in him, Lord, and you will not try him beyond what he can bear. I beg you, give him a sign that you are with him. Send your Mother to console him. Touch him with the knowledge of your love.

———

Letter to Jean Fox from Fr. Michael Shields

February 20, 2003

Dear Jean,

I want to tell you how I am experiencing Madonna House's deep call to support and care for priests.

I thank God from the bottom of my heart for my dear sisters. For Marie at a distance, who receives my rambling pain by e-mail and invests it with a sense of truth. For Miriam, who through her own suffering has come to a new depth of understanding and to a new wisdom and compassion that really astound me. For Sushi, for her kind hospitality and her incredible heart, which she has found anew in Magadan and gives to others in ever deeper ways.

I am so privileged to have Madonna House in my life, and I thank God for the strength of the prayers of all the priests and friends in Combermere. I know with all my heart that I would be spiritually dead without those prayers. Sitting at the table in Madonna House Magadan, I have found consolation in sharing tea with these women who hide in the heart of Jesus and love priests. I have found with them the peace that is beyond understanding and have become revived to fight again for the sake of souls—of mine, mostly.

I am a priest in every fibre of my being, and I will die a priest, on fire with Christ's love. But now I am suffering spiritually, so deeply that at times it leaves me numbed with pain. I go to bed in pain and rise in pain and live in it throughout the day, not because I want it, but because it is redeeming my poor soul.

Who really wants a cross that crucifies? And who can ever really imagine what the resurrection looks like? Only those who hang on to his promise and keep shouting from the tomb, "I believe you can do it in me," who do not try to crawl out of the tomb by their own strength, thus settling for just a few more moments of life resuscitated, but who instead keep trusting and praying for the grace to wait for a totally new reality that only God can create in the depths of one's soul.

He says, "Don't settle for a life resuscitated when you can have resurrection!" The first is just life as it has been; the other is a new life never known before. The price—death, the reward—life on high in Christ Jesus.

How God will bring forth his mighty work in one who feels like a useless floor rag remains a mystery. But he is life, even when we don't know where life can come from. He is hope, even when we say things have gone too far. He is love, even when we say there is too much war.

I am a priest, and in Madonna House I have advocates who honour what God has ordained as sacred and irrevocable. Yes, Satan may taunt me with his nasty half-truths, but my sisters remind me of *the* Truth and how the Truth has already won the victory.

I want you to know, Jean, that in one small apartment in northeast Russia, a priest is bowing before two women and their call, thanking God for all he is doing through them. They themselves suffer as they try to love each other in a supernatural way as sisters in the Lord. In their weakness they have truly become strong in Christ. Such a witness is a grace; such a witness is Christ himself.

Fr. Michael of the Heart of Jesus

March 5, 2003 – Ash Wednesday

Yesterday Sushi and I locked horns again. The point of the conflict was minor but I wouldn't let it go, and today I am tasting the ashes of my self-righteousness. I feel like the elder brother of the Prodigal Son. How did I get back there? What has happened to my heart?

Lent is a time for repenting of *my* sins, not for identifying the sins of others. A time for repenting and not for preaching about repentance. I should be fasting from criticism as well as from food!

COMBERMERE

March 25, 2003 – Feast of the Annunciation

The adjustment to Combermere seems harder this year. My anxiety is heightened by fatigue, the lack of a role, and the absence of anyone with whom I can really talk.

The solution? To anchor myself in the poustinia of my heart, to stand as a holocaust, and to claim my place at the bottom of the heap, at the foot of the cross, in the kingdom of the Beatitudes.

May 5, 2003

I keep catching myself trying to find a stance that will eliminate the inner pain. But we aren't talking about pain elimination; we're speaking of redemptive suffering! They are totally different realities.

Deep down I do trust God, but the surface continues to bubble and simmer. I obviously am not content to be little, and the old self dies harder than I want to admit. After five years with MS, I still seem to be at the very beginning.

The answer from which we all shy away: to stand in the pain and let it be; not to wallow in it, but not to seek an escape either. How difficult this is! We want to "have it together," or at the very least, to suffer elegantly.

A key, it seems to me, is to not resist. The victory consists in not letting the pain divide or isolate one, but in accepting and offering it with humility, and in willing that it become a force towards unity. This can only happen through prayer and through uniting oneself with Jesus' redemptive sacrifice.

Lord, help me to stay with you! My every instinct is to try to do it myself. And it's not even a matter of "how" to do it, but of living in you.

May 7, 2003

A new bishop, Kirill Klimovich, has been named for our diocese, replacing Bishop Jerzy. After a whole year without a resident Ordinary, the appointment comes as a relief. A citizen of Belarus, Bishop Kirill presumably will not be subject to visa restrictions.

My goddaughter Galya Knol, along with her mother and son, has been living in our apartments while we have been gone. They are in the process of renovating their own apartment and asked if they might stay on until Sushi returns

from her holidays after the Directors' Meetings. Since I will
be back in Magadan before Sushi, I suggested the following living arrangement: that she and her mother continue to
use the bedroom in Apt.19 and that we offer fifteen-year-old
Alyosha the kitchen-bedroom in Padre Pio's. This will give
him the privacy he craves, while freeing the living room for
common use. And I will have my beloved poustinia room in
St. Theresa's.

MAGADAN

The joke was on me.

I flew into Magadan on June tenth, and Igor, our parish driver,
met me at the airport. When we pulled up in front of our building,
Galya was outside, waiting to welcome us. "Where shall I put your
bags?" Igor wanted to know. Before I could tell him to bring them to
St. Theresa's, Galya said, "Apt. 19."

I soon discovered why. It had seemed logical to her that her
family move into St. Theresa's, freeing the main apartment for my
use and for those who are used to coming there to visit. They had
already transferred their belongings, including the cat. And while
this was undoubtedly the most practical arrangement, I didn't know
whether to laugh at the Lord's sense of humour or cry at being
evicted from my own room!

I was grateful that God gave me the grace to take it in stride, and
in the end, I was grateful for the opportunity of living side-by-side
with this Russian family. Galya's mother insisted on cooking for us
all, even though she worked as a night watchman at a school. We
all had different schedules and ate whenever it was convenient. It
frequently worked out that Galya and I had supper together. During
these weeks, we became real friends.

At the end of June, the Knols moved back to their own home,
and Galya helped me get ours ready for Sushi's return. Ira, the student who had helped us the previous summer with cooking and
housework, was available again this year.

For the past two years, a group of teenage girls from the parish
had been meeting with Sushi at our house for prayer and sharing.
Sushi was accompanying several of them on pilgrimage to Medjugorje

for three weeks in August, and during this time, she wanted Ira to whitewash the kitchen ceiling. .

I didn't know anything about whitewashing ceilings—but I did know that in Magadan, everything usually turned out to be much more complicated than anticipated. Just as I feared, the projected three-day job turned into a ten-day marathon.

Scraping away the loose ceiling plaster revealed gaping holes that needed to be filled. Galya, who was only supposed to advise Ira, spent an entire week of her holidays helping her scrape and cement. Providentially, Ilya, one of the youths in the parish came by to say hello and offered his services. I couldn't scrape or whitewash, but I cooked for the young workers, using the stove in Padre Pio's while the kitchen was inaccessible. I washed dishes in the bathtub, did the laundry and ironing, watered the plants in all three apartments, and kept things in order the best I could. In order to free Ira for the ceiling project, I took on all the work she had been hired to do for me!

The evening before Sushi's return, Ilya and Ira finished the last coat of whitewash and spent another two hours cleaning through the apartment. They were so eager to please Sushi—and they succeeded.

At the beginning of September, Liza returned. Sushi and I were quite impressed with the progress she had made in Russian. Katia was in Combermere, slated to join us after the new year.

Ten years in Magadan

<u>September 14, 2003 – Exaltation of the Cross</u>

Though I tried to hide it, at the heart of today's tenth anniversary celebration, there was for me an aching sense of emptiness. No one was present with whom to share the memories of the foundational years. Neither Alma nor Marie was here, and talking to them on the phone—Alma could hardly speak through her tears—only intensified the sense of absence.

Fr. Michael himself was out of the country renewing his visa. When we first discussed this anniversary with him, he suggested postponing it until his return. But because the offering of our lives in atonement for the camps is such a deep

element of our vocation here, we were reluctant to disassoci-
ate our celebration from the actual feast of the Holy Cross.

The Sunday Mass should have been an opportunity to
celebrate with our parish family, but the congregation was
unusually small. Almost none of the people to whom we are
close were present. Only a few had been in the parish when
we arrived in 1993; others had moved away, had not yet
returned from summer holidays, or were doing something
else.

These lacunas were more noticeable to me than to the
others. In every other way, the celebration was full of joy
and genuine appreciation for Madonna House. Fr. David
was simple and sincere as he thanked us for our life and our
prayer, for our support of the priests and the parish. The
reception after Mass was heart-warming.

Our afternoon open house was attended by old friends
and new, including some non-parishioners and several of
our neighbours. The presence of so many young people was
particularly delightful. People toured the ten-panel photo display into which I had poured so much effort—each panel por-
traying the events of one year—and then sat down to refreshments. Sushi's idea of setting up the fifteen-minute Madonna
House Magadan video* in the bedroom helped keep things
flowing. As a team, the three of us moved remarkably well.

Galya Knol and two of her friends found themselves a
corner and spent the afternoon deep in conversation. When
they explained to us, "We feel like this is our own home," I
had a flashback to our house blessing in 1993, when Marie
said to our guests, "This house belongs to Our Lady, which
means it belongs to all of you!"

Let it be, Miriam. Stand in your pain and know I am working.

---

* *The Silence of the Poustinia.* When the church opening in 2002 was videotaped for
the Catholic TV station in Novosibirsk, at our request a video of Madonna House
was also made.

COMBERMERE

March 20, 2004

I've just returned from seeing Mel Gibson's film, *The Passion* with Jean Fox. She drove, and we talked for the whole hour-and-a-half trip to Pembroke.

She said, "I understand everything you are saying. But at this point in history, the only thing that is going to change the world is for people to stand in the suffering and offer it."

Her implication was clear. Our situation in Magadan is the cross God is offering me. On my acceptance of the suffering depends infinitely more than I can begin to realize.

This is the heritage Catherine has given us. Foreign as it is to our Western mentality, we are being challenged as a community to take up the cross.

I told her "yes". We went in to watch the film. When it was over, there was nothing more to say.

April 6, 2004

Jean Fox died this morning. Two days ago, as she was getting dressed for the Palm Sunday Mass, she suffered what the doctors called a "catastrophic stroke" and never regained consciousness.

The preceding Friday Liza and I had spent over an hour with her, working out a plan for Liza to participate in the Russian publications. Jean looked exhausted, but she was as gracious as ever, and the time was blessed.

How I had resisted Sushi's insistence that I come to Combermere at this time of year! By the mercy of God, I am here.

I am too numb to write more.

April 17, 2004 – Easter Saturday

This is the first time since Catherine's death that I have been in Combermere for a funeral. Grieving together with the family brings a grace and a consolation of its own.

For each of the women, as well as for many of the men and priests, Jean was the one who knew our deepest heart, affirmed its goodness, and helped us to recognize God's presence in our lives.

When I opened the Scriptures today, the pain hit me afresh, and I couldn't go any further.

It will be better when I return to Magadan and get back to work. I feel as if Jean has given me a mission to carry the cross. But without her, there will be an added dimension of solitude.

MAGADAN

"The blood of martyrs is the seed of the Church"

At the end of June, Sushi, Katia, Liza, and I regrouped as a foursome. We quickly found ourselves drawn into the preparations for consecration of the new church.

The event was particularly significant in that it was happening in a city whose existence was synonymous with the gulag. The blessing of the Martyrs' Chapel on the evening *before* the church consecration was a potent reminder that the suffering and faith of the prisoners in the slave labour camps of Kolyma were the real foundations of the parish.

The prayer service began in the main church in the presence of a congregation swelled by forty or fifty camp survivors. Our own bishop, Kirill Klimovich, was joined by the new archbishop of Anchorage, Bishop Joseph Werth of Novosibirsk in western Siberia, and Bishop Clemens Pickel, whose diocese covered the southern European portion of Russia.

During the service, Bishop Werth spoke of his 1991 visit to the notorious uranium mining camp in Butyguchag, northwest of Magadan. "I looked out from the tiny window of the barracks and tried to imagine what a priest-prisoner might be thinking and praying," he recounted. "This priest would have known that 'the blood of martyrs is the seed of the Church.' He would have prayed in the hope that a time might come when the Church would be reborn, and believers would once more be able to freely practice their faith. We are now witnessing the fulfillment of this prayer," he concluded, and his voice broke.

Bishop Werth comes from a family of Volga Germans, descendents of the German immigrants invited to Russia by Catherine the Great in the late eighteenth century to form farming communities. During World War II, Stalin exiled the entire German community to Siberia and Central Asia. With only the belongings they could carry, the bishop's grandparents and their family were summarily herded into cattle cars and transported to Kazakhstan. There, in midwinter, the passengers were dumped on the frozen steppes and left to fend for themselves, digging underground shelters to shield themselves from the elements, eating roots, and begging what food they could from villagers. Hundreds died. The bishop's grandfather was sent to Kolyma. This history is seared on his heart.

Carrying vigil lights and small metal crosses, the congregation processed to the adjoining Martyrs' Chapel. Small and square, with a high ceiling and deeply-set windows, the chapel was dominated by two large icons, the work of the same Moscow artist who painted the icons in the main church. One icon depicted the twentieth century martyrs of Russia. Its uniqueness lay in the representation of both Catholic and Orthodox clergy, the former identified by their mitres, the latter by the *klobuk*, a black cylindrical head covering covered by a veil hanging down the shoulders and back. The second icon, similar in style, was a new composition called "The Martyrs of Kolyma." Here confessors of the faith, their names engraved in the gold nimbus above their heads, surrounded Our Lady. Stretching into the distance were ranks of unnamed martyrs.

"Before thy Cross, we bow down in worship, sovereign Lord, and thy holy Resurrection we glorify," we sang as men and women in a seemingly endless file, many of them moving laboriously or leaning on canes, placed on the altar their crosses and lit candles in memory of friends and relatives who had died in the camps. The crosses would later be affixed to the polished black granite stones lining the lower portion of the chapel walls.

The following day—the day of the actual consecration—was sunny and hot, at least by Magadan standards. The church was packed with parishioners, invited guests, friends, strangers, and many of the camp survivors who had been present the preceding evening. Once again, Bishop Kirill was the main celebrant.

Our new bishop was a short, stocky man with reddish hair, deep blue eyes, and a rare smile, which, when it appeared, lit up and transformed his face. He had been born in Kazakhstan, where his ethnic-Polish family had been deported. When he was still a child, they moved back to Belarus. Ordained to the priesthood in Poland, he became pastor of a parish in Belarus and then auxiliary bishop of Minsk. Last year, when it became evident that Bishop Mazur would not be permitted to return to the diocese, Bishop Kirill was appointed as his successor. This was his first visit to Magadan.

We were all struck by the passion that poured forth from this bishop's heart as he began his homily. Preaching in a resonant voice from behind the altar, using neither microphone nor notes, he emphasized that the faith that had sustained the Christians in the camps was the same faith that sustained and guided us today, enabling us to face without fear an uncertain future. The same Christ who suffered with those in the camps was with us now, filling us with hope and confidence.

The bishop raised one essential point that had not been addressed the preceding day: *the need to forgive*. He challenged the camp survivors to forgive their tormentors. He called for wives of alcoholics to forgive their husbands, for children and young people to forgive their parents, and for all of us, without exception, to seek reconciliation with those who had wronged or hurt us. He spoke strongly and unequivocally, and people listened.

Three strong images remained with me from the actual consecration: Bishop Kirill, the sleeve of his alb rolled up above the elbow, assiduously rubbing holy oil over every centimetre of the white marble altar; the four vested bishops climbing up and down chairs to reach and anoint the twelve crosses mounted on the walls in memory of the twelve apostles; and finally, two of our parish women wiping the oil from the altar and setting the banquet table of the Lamb with coordinated gestures and exquisite reverence.

Before our eyes, cement and steel, marble, stone, and wood were transformed by the Holy Spirit into the house of God.

After dinner at the parish that evening, four staff workers accompanied three Russian bishops and one American archbishop to

Madonna House for tea and dessert. We had anticipated this gathering as a unique opportunity to acquaint the bishops with our apostolate, but as it turned out, they were too tired and overloaded with the impressions of this very full day to absorb any more verbal input. They were overwhelmed with the very fact of being in Magadan.

And so, putting aside our own hopes for the evening, we responded to what really interested them—not our apostolate, but Kolyma itself. We brought out folders with articles about the gulag and maps with the locations of the numerous labour camps. Our library included many camp and prison memoirs. Especially fascinating was a book I'd just brought from Moscow, a large album of drawings and text by a Moldavian woman, vividly depicting her eighteen years of forced exile, prison, and internment in a labour camp above the Arctic Circle. Bishop Werth, in whose diocese most of this took place, exclaimed, "Every bishop in Siberia should have this book!"

Any Russian would have just given him our copy. I didn't. But Sushi offered it to Bishop Kirill, who stayed up reading it until two in the morning, unable to tear himself away from the saga. I ordered a copy for Bishop Werth through Raia and Volodya in Moscow.

Bishop Kirill's parting words to us remained in our hearts: "Your prayer is important here. Your presence is important. *Do the will of God. Only the will of God matters, not what anyone else thinks.*"

The Spirit is a-moving

In September Sushi and I attended a retreat on Lake Baikal, preached by Fr. Michael, for women religious of the diocese. On our return to Magadan, I wrote to Susanne Stubbs, who had succeeded Jean as Director of Women:

> Do you remember the song, "The Spirit is a-moving all over, all over this land"? Since attending the retreat for diocesan religious, this is the sense I have about our apostolate in the Irkutsk diocese and in Russia.
>
> The two retreats, one for the priests and one for the women, were well attended. Fr. Michael emphasized that we all are called to intimate union with God. He identified the obstacles we run into and suggested ways to overcome them.

It was a call to conversion, and I was moved to surrender my life to Christ on the cross at an even deeper level than before.

The ten nuns who joined Sushi and me for the women's retreat are all busy and overworked, and they drank up the opportunity to spend long periods in adoration, the prayer of the Church, and personal meditation. On the last evening, as we sat chatting, one of the nuns asked about poustinia, which had been mentioned during the talks. Sushi and I suddenly found ourselves the centre of attention. Some of the sisters had read *Poustinia* in Russian or Polish, and one of them makes a monthly poustinia. They all seemed hungry to touch God in this way.

At the priests' retreat the week before, the pastors of the two largest parishes in the diocese had remarked to Fr. Michael, "Madonna House has the spirituality for lay people." Fr. Antony Badura, head of the Claretians in Krasnoyarsk, added, "We *need* Madonna House!"

When Fr. Michael repeated this to us, my heart leapt. I heard it as a call to serve the diocesan Church specifically through the sharing of our Madonna House spirituality. I could easily see Katia and me going out in Lent or after Easter to talk with lay groups about Catherine's spirituality. The books already translated into Russian provide a foundation from which to work.

Susanne, this house has been through so much suffering! Marie, Alma, and Trudy have all paid a great price. My sense now is that these past five years have been a time of preparation, and God is beginning to reveal a new direction for Madonna House in Russia.

October 11, 2004

Sushi left yesterday to return to Combermere. Katia has been appointed LD *pro tem*. I know she will be graced.

She will be the fourth director I've had here in about as many years. It isn't easy to be under someone so much younger, both in age and in apostolic experience, but I thank

God for the trust and love that has grown between us this year. I am grateful for her sensitivity and her desire to serve. I may not always agree with her, but I am called to pray, communicate, support, and follow. Once again, the Spirit is calling me to littleness.

After our conversation last night, I felt the burden of carrying the apostolate slide from my shoulders. I felt Katia's grace of state, her peace and compassion, and the unity between us.

Praying last night before the Blessed Sacrament, my heart was wonderfully silent.

October 23, 2004

I had shown Katia the report I'd sent Susanne after Sushi and I returned from Lake Baikal. Last night we found ourselves discussing the possibility of doing some kind of presentation in Krasnoyarsk and possibly Irkutsk.

Katia was doubtful of her ability to speak publicly in Russian, but she said, "If you can carry it, I'll be happy to support you. I think I could learn a lot from you."

I felt like crying.

We have to talk it over with Liza and then ask Susanne. If she agrees, I will draft a letter to Fr. Antony Badura with our proposal. Since I will be leaving in a few weeks for my usual two-month stay in Combermere, nothing much can happen until I return. We'll take it step by step and see what God has in mind.

November 1, 2004 – All Saints Day

I have always looked for a role and then battled anxiety when I found myself hanging in the breach. But last week God pierced my fatigue and offered me a clear invitation. With Katia and Liza ably handling the day-to-day running of the house and apostolate, I am finally able to live within my limitations, serving in the ways I can, with my eyes on Christ—living for him, in him, through him. What freedom this is! Compared to this opportunity, who wants a role?

Lord, help me to stay in this reality. The spiritual life is not about "getting it together," but of letting my own constructs collapse so that I can perceive the infinitely more life-giving reality of existence in you.

I have learned that the times of greatest pain are the cradle of great blessings. No, emotions are not to be disregarded. They lead me to the spiritual reality—to repentance, trust, self-abandonment, freedom, and joy.

November 9, 2004

God gave me the strength to carry on for the time Sushi and I were alone together, but now I have a sense that the MS is taking its toll. At the retreat on Lake Baikal, I responded to an urge of the Spirit to offer myself at a new depth, to unite myself more fully with Christ on the cross. I knew it was from the Lord, for I couldn't have even conceived of it myself. I moved in the obedience of faith, knowing I was being pulled beyond my depth, but that he would be faithful.

This has been the underlying reality of the past month, in which Katia, Liza, and I have been together.

I'll probably return to Magadan after my stay in Combermere, but I have an intuition that it will not be for very long. Amazingly, this no longer upsets me. The only thing that is important is God's call, my trust in him, and his promise.

"Take up my yoke and learn from me, for I am meek and humble of heart, and I will give you rest. Yes, my yoke is easy, and my burden light." (Mt 11: 28-30).

"I am with you always; yes, to the end of time." (Mt 28:20)

Be Not Afraid

Monday before Ash Wednesday, February 7, 2005

Yesterday after Mass Katia and I stayed behind in the church to tidy up the songbooks. We ended up talking for almost an hour about how to cover the needs of the house while Liza is away in Combermere.

Katia's awareness and acceptance of my physical needs moved me deeply. I found myself admitting that I felt more handicapped than before I left last November. The tears in Katia's eyes told me I was in reality.

I just can't do it! I stretch myself beyond the edge of fatigue, an edge which keeps drawing closer than I want to recognize. I keep going until I can hardly move, until exhaustion grips not only my muscles but my whole nervous system, consuming what feels like my entire being. Then I don't sleep, I wake up exhausted, and it takes several days to get back into a normal rhythm.

I've never wanted to say, "I can't do it." Often I've been given the grace to move beyond what I thought possible. We have been so shorthanded for the past few years that often there has been no other choice. When Sushi and I were here alone, I grew out of the habit of "conserving my strength for the long haul," as Jean put it, and tried to respond to the needs I saw. I tried to give without reserve. It probably isn't an exaggeration to say the house would not have survived otherwise.

What is God saying to me now?

February 21, 2005

Fr. Michael has asked our friend Lyuda to begin collecting the stories of the camp survivors who are still in Magadan. I was delighted when she asked to come discuss this with me. Katia, however, had reservations about us getting involved with the church project. "I have to stop by the church this afternoon; I'll talk to Lyuda," she said.

I nodded, choking back my protest. I'd been looking forward to the opportunity to work with someone outside the house, and though we all love Lyuda, I rarely have a chance to be with her these days. But I can't use others to satisfy my desire for involvement—this is elementary.

This incident is a warning.

Living in truth means acknowledging, accepting, and offering the progression of the MS.

I think the time is approaching for me to leave Magadan.

———•••———

Letter to Marie Javora in Combermere

February 23, 2005

Dear Marie,

When I wrote the other day, I wasn't quite ready to face what God seemed to be saying. However, he has moved much more swiftly than I could have imagined. That same afternoon Katia and I found ourselves talking, and I felt pushed inwardly to tell her what had been coming to me about leaving Magadan. To our mutual amazement, God seemed to be saying the same things to her.

Monday in poustinia, as I was writing in my journal, realizations had begun to flow, as it were, from my pen onto the paper. The first, as I wrote to you, was that my own time in Magadan was drawing to a close. It wasn't a matter of being forced to accept this, but a quiet knowledge in my heart that it was so.

The next realization was that this has marked consequences for our apostolate in Magadan. I'd never considered it from this perspective. Of the three of us presently assigned to the house, Katia and Liza feel deeply called to Russia, but only I feel a specific call to offer my life here in Kolyma. "Feeling" isn't the right word. God is the one who places the desire in our hearts.

The call to the cross has always seemed to me the deepest meaning of our apostolic life in Magadan. It is the reality that has grounded us and given us strength to remain in this place where the spiritual battle is so particularly intense. It has brought us to the heart of Catherine's vocation to offer her life for the Church and priesthood.

The need for atonement will always be an essential part of our mandate in Russia. But since the MS has made this my particular "work" in the house, where does my departure leave us? What does God want for Madonna House in Russia?

The development of our apostolate in Magadan has been influenced by the situation of the Catholic Church in Russia, the particular nature of Magadan, and the nature of this parish.

Magadan is a small city, and because of the tensions with the Orthodox Church, our field of apostolic action is limited. Our relationships are primarily, though not exclusively, in the parish. The parish and our house grew up together. We worked behind the scenes, supporting both the priests and the laity, but refrained from taking positions of responsibility in order to keep our Madonna House identity and spirit. Fr. Michael has understood this; we have experienced with him a rare and God-given spiritual unity. Ours is one of the few Catholic parishes in this country to have an all-Russian lay staff.

Following the church consecration last summer, we have all felt the parish taking on new vitality. The church itself has become the focus of parish life. It is only natural that the teenagers who once met at our house should now hang around the church. When one of them recently broke up with his girl friend, he and his buddy came knocking at Fr. Michael's window after midnight. He came to his priest for consolation!

Fr. Michael and Fr. David have now been joined by a priest from Slovakia. The Daughters of Charity are seriously considering a foundation here. The parish is well staffed, and Fr. Michael has lots of ideas for the coming year.

Most of the people with whom we have had deeper relationships have moved away. This will continue, since anyone who can leave Magadan eventually does so. There will continue to be new parishioners, of course, but their spiritual needs can be met through the parish.

We are deeply loved. But have we worked ourselves out of a job? And while I believe that our Nazareth life itself has deep and transcendent value, my real question is, *have we more to give Russia than is possible here in Magadan?*

I think we do.

The Russian translations of Catherine's works are a vehicle for sharing our spirituality, but it is still impossible for people in other parts of the country to come and see how it is lived out. Magadan is too far away and prohibitively expensive, and those who do come are overwhelmed by Kolyma's history. We saw this last summer when the bishops came to our house after the church consecration and were much more interested in the material we had on the gulag than in the spirituality of our community.

And now a door is opening for us in Krasnoyarsk. Fr. Michael, returning from a diocesan meeting last week, told us, "Fr. Antony is really serious about a foundation there."

With all these factors suddenly converging and coming into focus, I am reeling from the impact.

My departure could be a turning point. We have to take it step by step, but it feels as if the Spirit is beginning to move.

As I said at the beginning, I hadn't intended to share these thoughts until I'd had a chance to digest them myself. However, it has helped me to clarify them by writing

In considerable fear and trembling, and with much love,

Miriam

Moving with the Spirit

February 25, 2005

Now that I have shared with Katia the thoughts I had written to Marie, it almost feels as if the possibility we've been discussing has already come to pass! If the situation is truly the way we see it, and not just a figment of our imaginations, it is hard to construe any other outcome.

As Katia said, Magadan is like the back door to Russia. However—one doesn't stand forever in the doorway.

February 28, 2005

The situation feels totally surrealistic. All of a sudden, it was as if we had closed Magadan and opened a new house in Krasnoyarsk all by ourselves—and we very nearly got caught!

When we finally got through to Fr. Antony by phone, we discovered he had never received our e-mail asking about the possibility of coming to give a talk in Krasnoyarsk. After we re-sent it, there was additional confusion: I had expressed our readiness to accept his "longstanding invitation," not realizing he meant a Madonna House mission and not just a visit. We hastened to clarify that we had no authority to even discuss the possibility until we'd communicated with our directors!

March 7, 2005

Katia and I both sent e-mails to Susanne, describing what was happening and what we thought God was saying. Ever since we have been waiting in a kind of void, unable to move until we receive her response.

Today the answer came: Susanne wants us to go to Krasnoyarsk to talk to Fr. Antony about opening a house there. It is a clear confirmation that we are listening to the Spirit.

Fr. Antony, when we phoned him, suggested we come after Easter to meet with him and the other Claretians and to give a talk to a group of lay people training to be diocesan catechists. We will have three hours for our presentation.

I wonder, is it physically realistic for me to think of doing this?

March 12, 2005

These days are excruciating. More and more, it seems as if our work in Magadan will draw to a close with my departure. I feel as if everything that was so familiar has suddenly been transformed by a death sentence. Never have I been so aware of people's love for us. They haven't an inkling of what may take place.

March 20, 2005

Archbishop Hurley has been in Magadan for the past week, accompanied by two Daughters of Charity of St. Vincent de Paul. They are hoping to return in the near future to begin working with the parish. When we told the archbishop of our plans, he was totally encouraging.

Yesterday evening, after a farewell dinner at the church for the archbishop and the sisters, I found myself chatting with Archbishop Hurley while the others were finishing the dishes. He asked me about poustinia, and to my horror, I found myself groping for words. It had been a long day, and I suddenly couldn't articulate the concepts on which my whole life was based. Just then Fr. Michael came in and began talking of his own experience with poustinia, which got me off the hook.

I was mortified.

To experience the tangible shrinking of my world, not only physically but intellectually, would be the most terrifying prospect of all, were it not for the fact that God has taught me that my intellectual capacities are not the essence of my being. Moment by moment, he has given me the light, the grace, the spiritual vision to accept the progression of this disease. He will continue to be with me at every step; I cannot get ahead of him. I place myself in his hands without reserve.

Lord, please give me the clarity and strength to do your will when we go to Krasnoyarsk next month. I trust you, Jesus. You are directing us.

Monday of Holy Week, March 21, 2005

I feel as if we are about to betray our people, who ask only that we be here with them. It isn't that we don't want to! But God is asking of us something else. No matter which way I turn, I cannot see us staying.

Help me to walk with you, Lord, during this week of your Passion. When we walk with you, in your will, we are united with everyone we love and carry, and our emotions too will be in place. Holy Mother of God, help us. No one is betraying anyone! Help us to stay with you, our hearts at peace, even while they are filled with pain.

Love and pain are different from sentimentality. The latter is centered on oneself, while the former are lived in, with, and through Christ. The difference between sentiment and passion is the Passion. Living what Christ asks me to live: *"Not my will, but thy will be done."* (cf. Lk 26:43)

Saturday of Easter Week, April 2, 2005

I asked Fr. Michael how to stand with God when I am trapped in the fatigue that envelopes me like a thick fog, isolating me and threatening to pull me into myself. He said I am learning the difference between a theology of suffering and the actual experience. "Don't try to *think* yourself into the cross," he warned. "Try invoking the Lord with short appeals and ejaculations. He will come to you."

I told him I can no longer touch the desire for the cross, that I've lost the cutting edge of the call. His suggestion: "Pray for the desire to desire."

Krasnoyarsk

Situated at the very centre of Siberia, halfway between Magadan and Moscow, with a population of almost a million, Krasnoyarsk had a totally different atmosphere than Magadan. Life here did not seem such a concentrated struggle for survival. As we met and talked with people in the two Catholic parishes, it seemed to us that here was a greater freedom to choose one's path, to try a vocation, to pursue one's dreams. There was hope. And there was interest in Madonna House.

Our Claretian hosts did everything possible to make us feel welcome. "We want you to feel at home, so that you will make this your home!" one of the priests told me with a broad smile.

The morning after our arrival we had a long talk with Fr. Antony, the superior of the Claretian community, who suggested that before making a definite decision, it might be good for some of us to spend a few months in the fall actually living in the city. As he seemed to be taking it for granted that I would be accompanying Katia, we told him about my impending departure.

I had assumed that I'd be able to stay in Russia until the end of the year, but now, suddenly, there was a timetable. I said, first in my heart and later to Katia, "I will go whenever it is best for the apostolate."

The effort flattened me.

During these days Katia's attention was intensely focused on the task at hand, on listening to the Spirit. She needed to be free to move without me, for even activities as simple as walking around the neighbourhood or accompanying Fr. Antony to the supermarket were beyond my capabilities. I was also aware of the need to conserve my energy for the talks I would be giving. The closeness in which we had lived during the preceding weeks gave way to an overwhelming loneliness, which I struggled to offer for Katia and the future of Madonna House in Russia.

We had been invited to introduce our community and share something of Catherine's spirituality with a small group of men and women studying to be diocesan catechists. The weekend session was being held in an apartment owned by the parish. When Katia and I joined them Sunday afternoon, they greeted us as if we had known each other for years.

Despite my trepidation, the presentation flowed easily. Telling the story of Catherine's life, I tried to convey how her obedience to the Spirit, her passionate desire to do God's will, and her embracing of pain as a way of "consoling the lonely Christ" had led to the development of an international lay apostolate. Next we showed the video in which interviews with Catherine were interspersed with footage taken at her funeral. The narration had been translated into Russian by Alvina and professionally dubbed. Catherine's human and spiritual charisma had been captured so well that the film had often been described as "anointed." This time, too, it left a deep silence and joy in the room.

After the tea break, I continued with an overview of Madonna House spirituality, using a small book of excerpts from Catherine's writings I had compiled and Alvina had translated.* We concluded with the fifteen-minute video about our house in Magadan, *Silence of the Poustinia*. I could feel the group responding.

When I asked Katia about her impressions of the afternoon, she responded dryly, "If the fact that two of them were crying when you said good-bye is any indication, I'd say it went quite well!"

From Krasnoyarsk Katia and I flew to Moscow. She continued to the Directors' Meetings in Canada, and I spent a few days with Raia and Volodya.

Two days before I was to leave for Magadan, Volodya was attacked by thugs near his home. He was hospitalized in critical condition, and I stayed an extra week to support Raia. Her gratitude was an irrefutable confirmation that presence is the most important gift I could offer.

The evening Volodya landed in the hospital, the phone never stopped ringing. Every time we picked up the receiver, we feared it would be a message that he had died, but each call came from someone offering prayers, concern, or help. Finally, after midnight, Raia said, "All Moscow is praying for him. The prayers are keeping him alive."

What an incredible woman she was! When he had been in intensive care for almost a week with no visitors permitted, she said to me, "I have to see him. He has to know that people love him."

---

* *God in the Nitty-Gritty Life,* Madonna House Publications, 2002.

MAGADAN

May 4, 2005

It is good to be back in Magadan. I am so grateful that Susanne gave me permission to stay here alone until Liza returns from Canada. I drink from the silence and solitude.

Yesterday evening I sat for a long while in the chapel. It was 10:30 P.M., and the light was just beginning to fade. It seems a long time since I simply sat in silence. A long time since that kind of silence has been *in* me.

There is no tangible apostolic activity just now. No demands from the outside. I know better than to try to justify my existence with activity. I am back to "being."

I can't touch "Russia." I'm not even touching our people here; no one is coming to visit. I can't touch the love that is in my own heart. Where all these realities once lived so intensely there is only quiet.

May 18, 2005

Katia phoned from Combermere to tell me that Marie will be returning with her at the end of June. They will go together to Krasnoyarsk for the initial reconnaissance period, not in October as we had thought, but in August. Liza will use those months to continue her Russian studies.

This means my departure date will also be moved up again. My first reaction, a sense of helpless victimization, was reinforced by the realization that my Moscow friends will still be away on holiday in August. I was tempted to give in to indignation and self-righteousness—"I should at least be able to say good-bye to my friends!" But that would be to impose conditions on what needs to be a wholehearted acceptance of God's will.

Russians do not expect life to bow to them. One does what one must. Did Stalin's victims have a chance to say good-bye? Not that there is any comparison with my own situation, but I can offer my frustration in their memory.

Put your hand to the plough and do not look back (cf. Lk 11:62).

*Lord, you made us to live in you, and I really believe it is possible.
Even our emotions are appeased when you become our focus.*

May 24, 2005

Liza is back!

Having let go of my departure date, having placed it in
the Lord's hands and embraced his will deep in my being, I
could almost leave at any moment.

Pondering this, it comes to me that:

1) When we really believe God's will is life-giving, we
can let him write the script for our lives. We can surrender
the need to control what happens to us. A big chunk of fear
falls away—the fear that we will die inwardly if this or that
condition isn't fulfilled.

2) Another big chunk of fear leaves us when we come to
accept suffering. Freed from the bondage of fear, we are able
to let God use us how and where he pleases.

"You will learn the truth, and the truth shall make you free." (Jn
8:31-3)

June 6, 2005

Last night I began reading Pope John Paul II's *Crossing
the Threshold of Faith*. In the very first chapter, he comments
on the theme that ran through his whole pontificate, "Be not
afraid."

Fear has always been my root sin. I have been praying for
courage, and at Pentecost this year, when we passed around
the basket with the gifts and fruits of the Spirit, to my amazement I drew "fortitude," the closest gift to it. "Fortitude" was
the gift and "love," the fruit.

June 27, 2005

When I went to OVIR today, I was told that there is no
way of knowing when my new residency card will be ready.
Since I can't leave until it is in my hand, I am thrown back
into a situation of open-ended trust and surrender.

I'd already composed the scenario of my departure, surrounded by my sisters and Fr. Michael. The one thing I'd

hoped for was to leave before the eventuality of the house closing became known. Now, anything can happen.

Lord, this is your script. I renounce my desire to write it. Help me to keep walking in this path of freedom. Holy Lady of Combermere, take my hand and help me run with you wherever you are hastening, like a little child trying to keep up with her Mother. Thank you, Lord, for helping me to recognize the bonds of fear. They are broken each time I surrender to your will in trust and confidence.

July 11, 2005

We have just learned that I can travel on my old residency card after all, which means we can proceed with our original departure schedule. Liza and I will fly to Moscow on August eleventh, and Katia and Marie to Krasnoyarsk on the seventeenth.

Fr. Michael suggested we tell the parishioners what we are doing "so they will have time to grieve."

Russians grieve well. It is something I have learned from them. They don't hide their emotions, and they have taught me that pain and tears can coexist with acceptance and surrender. With them it's not "either/or" but "both/and."

July 18, 2005

I may be spared, after all, the chalice of pain, a public suggestion that the house might close. Liza and I had prepared a draft in Russian of the announcement Katia planned to read at the Sunday liturgy, but early yesterday morning Susanne e-mailed Katia that she thought it was much too early to make any announcement. She feels we should take it step by step and not get ahead of God. Since nothing except my own departure has been definitely decided, we do not yet have to start saying good-bye.

July 20, 2005

I awoke early this morning and dozed, mourned, wept, and struggled. I am inside the pain. The pain of having MS, the pain of loneliness, limitation, isolation, and impending departure.

I cried out silently, "Where am I?"

Christ answered, *"You are with me."* I hide under his hand, within his heart. On the cross, yes, but today, in his heart.

I accept. I offer. Struck from yet another direction, I react anew, I fumble, I flail about in my heart. I call out, and his voice brings me again to stillness. Or is it faith that stills me so that I can hear his voice? It really doesn't matter.

His words empower me to stand still within the pain. I accept it. I offer it. I take another step forward. *Thank you, Lord.*

July 25, 2005

My inner storm seems to have subsided. Going to confession broke the emotional battle and sealed the chinks against temptations. Conversations with Katia and Marie broke the sense of isolation. Communication always helps restore my balance. *Thank you, Lord. Thank you for my sisters.*

Fr. Michael was unexpectedly gentle. "You have an open wound now, and every pinch of salt exacerbates it. It's understandable. Your call is to suffer for Russia, so what you have to do is to offer the pain."

Thank you, Lord, for the gift of Fr. Michael in my life. You have used him so powerfully to bring me to yourself, and you have protected me from becoming emotionally involved with him. What more could I have asked? I thank you for the understanding of the past few years, for these quiet graces in confession and at the times when I've gone to him for discernment. Again and again, his ability to put old truths into fresh formulations, his gift of clarity, his acceptance of reality, and his perception of your presence have reoriented me and given me new vigour, freedom, and confidence.

I already miss him. In faith I know you will soon be filling this ache with new life.

So I want now to let go of Fr. Michael. "Want?" I sense that you are asking me to do this. It is your will for me. You aren't asking me to break off a relationship or to cast him out of my life. As I look into your beautiful face on the Rublev icon, I understand that everything is truly in order, in a way I could never have imagined. I let go now—in love, in trust, and in deep, inexpressible gratitude.

"How can I repay the Lord for his goodness to me?
I will lift up the cup of salvation
And call upon the name of the Lord." (Ps 115: 13-14)

July 28, 2005

Yesterday I awoke early and found myself mentally composing a letter to Bronislava and Olga. It was the first time I had found words to express what was so deep in my heart, but I couldn't write it down right away, and I've lost the clarity.

Lord, if it is your will, bring it back. If there is anything I can give to these people, help me to do so!

What they have suffered has become my point of reference over the years, relativizing my own difficulties and helping me to bear and offer them. How many times, chafing against my confinement, has the thought of their imprisonment dissolved my discontent? How often, balking at the limitations of my life, have I been reminded of all that was summarily and forever swept away from them? Their suffering has given meaning to mine. To the extent that I can be faithful to what they have taught me, their suffering and the suffering of millions of others will not have been in vain.

Thank you, Lord, for the incredible gift of having shared my life with them.

July 31, 2005

Yesterday Katia asked me to delay the publication of *Dear Father,* Catherine's book about the priesthood, until we are more settled. I had forgotten that we had spoken of this back in April, and I had indeed charged ahead on my own. It is natural enough to want to see it through, but the publications are not "mine."

It is a call to surrender yet another area of my life here. Although I will continue to work in Combermere on the preparation and correction of translations, it is only logical that the organization be done in Russia. There really isn't any resistance in my heart; I can let the tears come. Pain hurts, but it can be borne. *I offer it, Lord, for the future of our spirituality in Russia.*

August 6, 2005

I woke up in the night and wept for all the love that is carrying me these days. I sat on the edge of the bed and prayed before the little icon of Our Lady, a gift to me from a friend in Canada, which I will give to Galya Knol when I leave. The flickering light of the vigil lamp illuminated Our Lady's face and cast the shadow of the wildflower bouquet against the wall behind.

I don't want to get mired in sentimentality, but neither do I want to protect myself from true emotion. As I prayed, it came to me with absolute certainty that God is now inseparable from the way I experience reality. This is new for me.

The farewell celebration at the church turned out to be everything I could have wished. I hadn't had time on Saturday to practice my speech, but when I awoke Sunday morning, I put it in God's hands and actually had confidence it would be all right.

The congregation was small, as often happened in summer when people were on holiday or out working in their gardens. All the youth were at World Youth Day in Cologne. Olga had asked to be excused from Mass in order to attend her son's birthday celebration, but Bronislava and other camp survivors were there. On my way up to the lectern, I decided not to use the notes in my pocket. My heart was full, and I decided to let it spill forth.

Fr. Michael, introducing me, said, "Miriam is truly my sister." He repeated it a second time: "Miriam is my sister." I think he couldn't find any more words, for he just motioned me forward.

I told them what I had learned from them. I told them how they had taught me, and all of us, what Gospel love and self-giving really look like. I told them their lives and their acceptance of suffering had prepared me to accept the cross of multiple sclerosis, and that this was why God had brought me to Magadan.

After I finished speaking, Fr. Michael presented me with "yet another cross," one of the crucifixes he had brought from the Church of the Holy Sepulchre in Jerusalem last winter. Katia came up swiftly to help me down the three steps from the lectern.

Bronislava was openly crying, as were others in the congregation. Galya Knol hugged me, exclaiming, "That was the best homily I've ever heard about the cross!" I was showered with gifts, and eventually we moved into the room where tea and a beautiful farewell cake were being served. Katia, Liza, and Marie had come the previous evening to help blow up fifteen balloons so that, in Galya's words, I "would be able to breathe some Magadan air when I get lonely!"

Farewells, photos, tears, embraces. *Thank you, Lord, for the extraordinary privilege of being loved by these people.*

August 9, 2005

In a few days, I will be leaving Magadan. God has been so incredibly good to me that this step, which I feared for so long, has come with a gentleness I could never have anticipated.

God brought me to Russia that I might learn how to love and how to suffer. I can't imagine what I would be like, had I not come to this place. What I have lived here has become an indelible part of me.

One era comes to an end; another begins. After twenty years in France and Russia, and after having lived all but two of my thirty-three years of apostolic life in our various field houses, I am returning to Combermere and embarking on a new adventure.

THE JOY OF THE CROSS

(Adapted from an article published in Restoration, *January 2002)*

My paperback Jerusalem Bible has fallen apart. I've tried pasting it and taping it, and at this point, it's held together by a thick rubber band. I could replace it, but I can't quite bring myself to do so. Since Bibles shouldn't be thrown out, I would have to burn the old one, and each time the thought passes through my mind, I remember that not very long ago, a Bible was such a scarce and treasured item in Russia that people copied out passages by hand.

For twelve years I lived in Magadan—a northeastern Russian city that was once the administrative center for the Kolyma gulag system. For twelve years my outer and inner life was lived in the shadow of the camps. I have been haunted by the hundreds of thousands of lives that were shattered or buried there.

Part of the mandate for our Madonna House foundation in Magadan was to atone for the evil perpetrated in these camps. Pondering its personal application, I came to realize that an unbreakable link has been forged between the meaning of my own life and the lives that were sacrificed for no apparent purpose at all.

In Magadan the meaning of life and sacrifice never struck me as a subject for abstract discussion. There the mystery of the cross and resurrection was a tangible reality, illuminating not only the past, but also the continuing struggle to deal with the contradictions and hardships of daily existence.

My years in Magadan have seared me with the knowledge that ultimate meaning cannot lie in anything one can lose. It cannot be found in possessions, relationships, works, or health—all these were brutally stripped from the camp victims, for whom past and present dissolved in the ongoing battle to survive just one more day. I too must find my meaning in the present moment.

Our lives do not belong to us. Like the talents in the parable, they are entrusted to us that we might invest them with love and return them in gratitude, each moment of each day, to the Giver. "We offer you your own, from what is your own, in all, and for the sake of all" (from the Byzantine liturgy).

How we feel, physically or emotionally, has nothing to do with it. Whatever the content of a day or a moment offered to the Father, he accepts it and transforms it, through the power of Christ's sacrifice, into saving grace for the whole world. We have nothing to lose because nothing was ours in the first place—nothing but God's love, freely given and poured out on the cross.

The cross of Jesus Christ has been planted very concretely in my own life through the illness of multiple sclerosis. God prepared me for this by bringing me to Magadan. There he opened my heart to the love and suffering of those we had come to serve, but who gave us infinitely more than we could ever give to them. Gradually we realized that the only way we could stand with them was to offer ourselves for their sake.

In Russia, as one of our friends recently reminded me, everything is lived to the extreme. The cross is the extreme—but obvious—consequence of the desire to love.

Since no one except masochists and great saints actively seeks suffering, when we accept the suffering that comes to us, we can know we are fulfilling God's will and not our own. In accepting suffering, we can give it to him. In this way, what was a result of original sin becomes our free participation in Christ's saving work of love.

It is hard to put into words, but this is what unites me to the martyrs of Kolyma. I feel a responsibility towards them to accept my own difficulties rather than fight them, and to let these difficulties bring me to Christ and unite me to his sacrifice. To the extent that I do this, I am affirming the value of their suffering. If I flee the cross, if I deny its life-giving power, it is as if I betray those who could not flee.

In the Judeo-Christian tradition, "remembering" is a sacred obligation. "Let us remember and never forget: once we were slaves in Egypt, and the Lord delivered us with a strong hand and an outstretched arm," reads the Jewish Passover ritual. The same Lord tells us at each Mass, "Do this in memory of me." The Russian hymn for the dead is called *Vechnaya pamyat*—"Eternal Memory."

When we consciously live our lives in history—something that is rare in our modern civilization—those who have gone before us are part of our present. When we live in God, we are one with both the living and the dead in the Communion of Saints.

To live in the shadow of the camps is, ultimately, to live in the light of the Resurrection, where the robes of the martyrs are washed clean by the blood of the Lamb, where night is abolished, and the light of the Lord God shines forever.

This is the reality that transforms our whole life, freeing us from fear and illusion to seek the treasure our hearts most desire. This is the joy of the cross and the hidden treasure of Magadan.

Other Books from Madonna House Publications

Catherine Doherty:

Beginning Again
Bogoroditza
Catherine Doherty – Essential Writings
Dear Father
Donkey Bells
Fragments of My Life
God in the Nitty Gritty
Grace in Every Season
In the Footprints of Loneliness
In the Furnace of Doubts
Living the Gospel without Compromise
Not without Parables
On the Cross of Rejection
Poustinia
Sobornost
Soul of My Soul
Stations of the Cross

Eddie Doherty:

A Cricket in My Heart
Gall and Honey
Matt Talbot
Splendor of Sorrow
Tumbleweed

Visit: www.madonnahouse.org/publications
for a full catalogue